In Praise of
The Baby Sle...

Life changing

Amber

"This book has literally changed my life. Jam-packed full of helpful information, different approaches and general support. My only regret is that I did not buy this sooner. My house, baby and myself are so much more happy now we sleep all night and are in the best routine."

Easy-to-read advice, good fonts and simple, to-the-point paragraphs

Sally Hall

"Very helpful advice, which has given me confidence as a first-time mum into settling my baby. He is four months old, and successfully self-settling and sleeping through the night, which this book has given me assurance to do. It's easy to understand, with short snappy paragraphs, not too overwhelming and pocket sized."

A miracle book

Louise

"Cannot recommend this book enough, it is concise and set out in a way that it can be used as a reference for each stage of baby's life. Bought one for my friend's baby shower and everyone at our baby massage group has a copy. Within a few days of reading it my son was in a sleep routine; my friends also found this with their babies."

Brilliant book – would highly recommend

Emma

"I would highly recommend this book – it's really helped my four-month-old baby establish a good nap routine and has so many brilliant tips on settling. It's very practical and not too overwhelming – very readable for a busy mum!"

A must for first-time parents

Mrs CP2

"Short, sweet and practical. Ideal for when you are sleep deprived as it's delivered in easy-to-read, bullet-point-style language. I read it before my son was born and stuck with it. Best parenting book by far."

This has changed my life

Louisa

"This is amazing!! I was at the end of my tether with my baby's sleeping. Every day was a battle to get him to nap, which meant he spent the whole day tired and grumpy and scratching his face to bits. I thought I would have a long battle on my hands, but it's already working after a couple of days. He napped in his crib for the first time ever!"

Easy to read, guilt-free and effective!

Rosie

"Fantastic book. All the other sleep books just filled me with dread and guilt about how wrong I was doing things. This book is simple to read, gives you multiple options, which are actually realistic rather than super precise and prescriptive, and most importantly the methods work!"

An Hachette UK Company
www.hachette.co.uk

Vie Books, an imprint of Summersdale Publishers Ltd
Part of Octopus Publishing Group Limited
Carmelite House
50 Victoria Embankment
LONDON
EC4Y 0DZ
UK

www.summersdale.com

Printed and bound in Poland

P. 34–35 SIDS information has been reproduced with kind permission of The Lullaby Trust.

ISBN: 978-1-80007-875-8

Substantial discounts on bulk quantities of Summersdale books are available to corporations, professional associations and other organizations. For details contact general enquiries: telephone: +44 (0) 1243 771107 or email: enquiries@summersdale.com.

Disclaimer
The information given in this book should not be treated as a substitute for qualified medical advice. Neither the author nor the publisher can be held responsible for any loss or claim arising out of the use, or misuse, of the suggestions made or the failure to take medical advice. The case studies and quotes included in this book are based on the real experiences of individuals and families, however, in some cases, names have been changed to protect privacy. Although there is a move towards a more gender inclusive language, for the purposes of this book, the term breastfeeding is used throughout.

THE
BABY SLEEP
GUIDE

Practical Advice to
Establish Positive Sleep Habits

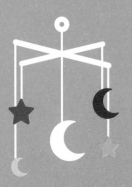

Stephanie Modell

Inspired by my children:
Alexander, Evangeline and Maxwell

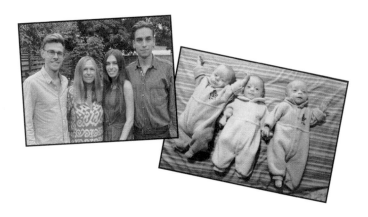

Contents

FOREWORD
to first edition
(March 2015)

By Jill Irving

RN (adult) RN (child) RM RHV JP

Almost 40 years ago when I became a health visitor, I thought lack of sleep was what happened after a late night out with friends. I had little concept of what any parent with a young sleepless child may be enduring until I became a parent myself.

My first son was born during the mid 1980s and I had been a health visitor for eight years by the time his non-sleeping brother arrived. I was meant to be supporting parents who were struggling with their own sleep-challenged babies, but I found it difficult to cope with even the simplest daily tasks in my own life.

For many years the only professional sleep advice recommended was controlled crying or – for those who were desperate – medication. Yes, for many years health professionals were recommending prescribed medication for children as young as 6 months old!

As hard as it may seem, it has only been since we've reached the twenty-first century that sleep problems among babies and young children have been acknowledged to be an increasing and serious problem.

Before this, parents were led to believe that it was normal for their babies and young children to regularly take hours to settle and spend hours awake each night. Parents were expected to get on with it as best they could, with virtually little or no support.

In 2012, a major online sleep survey by Mumsnet of 11,000 parents with children aged 0–10 years found that more than half had children waking at night; nearly a quarter of parents said their relationship with their partner had suffered; and almost a third said they felt regularly sleep deprived and exhausted. Without doubt this is a serious issue.

Research has also told us that directly or indirectly, lack of sleep can affect families by increasing the risk of postnatal depression, domestic violence and harm to children, separation and divorce rates, road traffic accidents, and affect work performance.

Thankfully, sleep consultants like Stephanie Modell are beginning to change parents' lives. Even better, Stephanie has produced this wonderfully simple-to-follow evidence-based guide for all those involved with babies and young children. Even if you are tired and exhausted, Stephanie gently leads you through each stage so that you gradually feel you are taking back some control of your life.

If you are expecting your first baby, buy this book now. If you are a parent struggling with a night-owl, buy this book now. If you are an excited grandparent to be or just about to go to a girlfriend's or relative's baby shower, ditch the cute booties and buy this book instead. This will be the best gift you could buy any potential parent.

Every health professional working with babies and young children should have at least two copies of this book in their office, as once they've lent out the first copy they'll never get it back!

Jill Irving

Jill Irving has been a practising health visitor for almost 40 years. She is an expert panellist for babycentre.co.uk.

Introduction

There are hundreds of sleep books available, but many contradict each other, and some are long and wordy and can make sleep a very complicated subject. My aim is to offer something different. I want to show you that sleep is not a difficult topic and that, by introducing positive sleep habits early on, you can minimise sleep problems later. I want you to discover that a well-rested baby is a contented baby. I'm not going to promise that I can get your baby to sleep for 12 hours a night at 12 weeks old. Babies do wake at night, this is nature's way of keeping them safe, but you can help them to sleep well with some gentle guidance, by following their own body rhythms and encouraging them to self-settle.

This book is not about 'training your baby to sleep'. Sleep is an automatic behaviour triggered by the build-up of sleep pressure. Foetuses sleep *in utero* with no learning involved. However, falling asleep in response to external (the carer's) cues rather than internal biological ones is a learned behaviour, so helping your baby to discover their own way of settling is a fundamental step in encouraging them to sleep through the night. By establishing positive sleep habits early on, sleep training should NEVER be necessary!

It's hard to absorb everything you are told and all that you read, particularly when you are tired and hormonal, so my intention is to provide you with the essential information, rather than an exhaustive book about sleep. Knowledge is empowering. I believe that if you understand the basic biology of sleep, you are much less likely to experience sleep problems with your baby. As a maternity nurse and mother of triplets, my advice is gleaned from professional experience as well as first hand when helping my own children to sleep through the night.

I will guide you through responsive, gentle parenting techniques that emphasise the importance of nurturing your baby and always responding to their needs, while gradually encouraging a little sleep independence. I will never suggest that you leave your baby to cry alone or to deprive a hungry baby of food.

When you are pregnant you receive mounds of information about what to expect with regard to the actual birth and what will follow, but the feedback I receive from parents is that postnatal information regarding sleep is lacking. The aim of this book is to fill that gap, with easy-to-read, accessible information on what is sometimes perceived to be the most difficult part of being a parent.

If possible, I highly recommend that you read this book during pregnancy and again in the early weeks.

If I could only say one thing!

If I could only say one thing to new parents it would be that there is no right or wrong way to parent your baby. If what you are doing works for you then you are doing the right thing for you and your family. However, if your older baby continues to wake many times during the night and it's affecting you and your family in a negative way then I will try to help you to make positive changes to encourage your baby to sleep for longer periods. Sometimes just making small tweaks to your routine can dramatically improve your baby's sleep without the need for further intervention.

If you would like to establish positive sleep habits from the start the first thing to work on is feeding. Whether you are breast- or bottle-feeding there is a strong correlation between feeding and sleeping. A hungry baby is unlikely to sleep well so, in the early weeks, this needs to be your primary focus.

A newborn's sucking reflex is strong, and allowing them to satisfy their sucking needs at this time will help you to establish an adequate and stable milk supply, if you choose to breastfeed. Breast milk also contains a range of hormones that have a soporific effect on babies and will induce sleep, especially during the early weeks when your baby sleeps in short but regular sleep cycles for optimal development.

However, the most common problem I come across as a sleep consultant is babies over 6 months old who have never learnt to fall asleep without a breast or bottle in their mouths, which in turn causes frequent night-time waking.

If your baby can only get to sleep in this way, they will be unable to self-settle and, in the longer-term, will be totally dependent on feeding to sleep. As they get older they will not have the ability to return to sleep at points during the night-time sleep cycle where they naturally wake. This often results in frequent waking and they will need to be nursed or fed back to sleep again.

It can be very hard to reverse a habit that may have been established for 6–12 months or more. This can cause a lot of unnecessary stress and sleep deprivation for both the baby and the parents, so I believe that it is better to gently encourage a baby to self-settle from a young age by introducing alternative sleep cues. This does not mean just putting them in their cot and expecting them to fall asleep. I will guide you through gentle and responsive techniques to encourage sleep.

There is no right or wrong way to parent.

Parenting styles

I work with families that have a variety of different parenting styles and I adapt sleep solutions to suit each family. It is really important you use sleep techniques that you feel comfortable with.

There are a number of publications covering two conflicting methods of parenting. One of these advises the development of a routine with a sometimes rigid feed and sleep schedule, as encouraged by Gina Ford in *The Complete Sleep Guide for Contented Babies and Toddlers*. The other is known as close proximity or attachment parenting, as described by William and Martha Sears in *The Attachment Parenting Book*.

Parenting to a strict clock-based schedule may work for some babies, but because all babies are unique one schedule cannot work for everyone. Within the realms of 'average sleep needs' and 'average sleep cycles' there can, of course, be great disparity. A baby's requirements will also differ depending on how they feed, their ability to feed efficiently, their health and tolerance to their milk feeds. If a mother is breastfeeding, her milk production will also play a factor in how often her baby needs to feed. For so many reasons, including our wonderful uniqueness, prescriptive clock-based parenting cannot work for all.

On the other hand, attachment parenting is completely baby-led, with an emphasis on closeness and responsiveness. The baby is carried in a sling or pouch throughout the day (frequently referred to as 'baby wearing') and parents, or often just the mother, bed share with the baby at night, allowing the baby to breastfeed as frequently as they wish, day and night.

Guidelines on bed sharing vary from country to country and, when I wrote the first edition of *The Baby Sleep Guide*, the UK guidelines stated that bed sharing should be avoided for safety reasons. However, the most recent research suggests that a high number of parents bed share anyway, either by choice or through desperation. There are a number of factors that must be taken into consideration and bed sharing should not be practised if any of them are applicable. These factors include: a premature or low birth weight baby; a parent who is a smoker or has consumed alcohol or drugs; sleeping with a baby on a chair or a sofa; or having loose covers or pillows in the bed that could cover the baby's head or cause them to overheat. Professor Helen Ball and her team at the Durham Infancy & Sleep Centre have published many papers on bed sharing and how to bed share as safely as possible. There is excellent information on their website: basisonline.org.uk.

Although there is a lot of information available on attachment parenting there is a lack of guidance on weaning your child from this close-proximity dependence, which can be a particular problem for working parents. For this reason, if you choose to bed share, I would strongly advise that you also encourage your baby to sleep independently (but in the same room as you) in their cot or Moses basket for some daytime naps. Once your baby is 8–9 months old and on the move it can be a real problem if they can only fall asleep when bed sharing with you. You may end up having to go to bed at 7 p.m. with your baby in order to get them to sleep and you may have to lay down with them for all naps if they do not know how to go to sleep in any other way.

Parenting today can seem wildly polarised: breast versus bottle; purées versus baby-led weaning; routine versus attachment, whereas in real life a lot of parents or carers find a healthy balance between the two opposing styles. I encourage you to go with the flow in those first few precious weeks while you recover from the huge journey of birth, getting to know your baby and establishing feeding, whether it be breast or bottle. I then aim to bridge opposing attitudes by advocating a blend of common sense, gentle guidance, practical advice and a lot of love.

I don't believe you need to make a choice as to whether to follow attachment parenting or a structured style of parenting. As parents, of course you want a securely attached child, and to achieve this you need to nurture a strong parent–child connection by meeting their physical, mental and emotional needs.

There is a middle ground, where you can have the best of both by following your baby's rhythms and cues to connect the bridge between nurture and structure, by encouraging some sleep independence and adopting a flexible routine.

Part One:

NEWBORN AND THE EARLY WEEKS

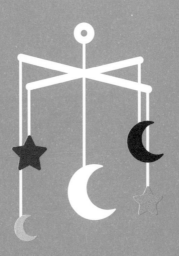

1. Realistic expectations

As well as getting prepared practically, it's really useful to prepare yourself mentally for parenthood. The reality is that from the birth, life will change and you may have periods of disturbed sleep for some years to come. Even if your baby sleeps through the night from 12 weeks old, they are likely to have regressions, which may be caused by developmental leaps, teething, illness, nightmares or separation anxiety.

Also, one parent's definition of sleeping 'through the night' might be that their baby does a 5-hour stretch, while another's may be a 10–12-hour stretch, so try not to compare your baby with others. I will give you all the tools to help your baby to sleep well, gently guiding them into learning how to self-settle. However, there are no hard-and-fast-rules here – every baby is different and, at the end of the day, they will sleep through the night when the time is right for them.

2. Visitors

Following the birth of your baby or babies, think about restricting your guests for a few days, or even a couple of weeks, and enjoy this special time without the stress of entertaining visitors.

You cannot overestimate how exhausting giving birth can be. Couple the physical effects with hormonal changes and the huge impact your child/children will have on your life – expect to be tired! This is your time for nesting, cuddling up with your new baby and partner, and bonding with each other.

3. Baby's first night at home

Babies are often very sleepy for the first night, when you're likely to be in hospital with help and support nearby. By the second or third night, babies sometimes start to realise that they are no longer in the warmth of the womb being lulled to sleep by a heartbeat and gentle, swooshing sounds, at which point they may suddenly find their voice. This can be worrying if you're a first-time parent, but your baby just needs cuddles and reassurance.

If you are breastfeeding, they may wish to feed constantly for comfort. This is a normal pattern of behaviour and will help to stimulate your milk supply – but be careful to get a good latch every time to avoid damaging the nipples. 'Latch' refers to how your baby is attached to the breast when feeding and is also known as 'a good attachment'. If you're bottle feeding, you may need to give small regular feeds.

4. Skin-to-skin contact

Offering skin-to-skin contact helps a baby to adjust to life outside the womb. It's calming and soothing, and can give your baby the comfort and reassurance they are craving. Baby is stripped down to a nappy and placed on either parent's bare chest, where they will hear the comforting sounds of your heartbeat as well as experience the warmth and comfort of your skin. It provides multiple benefits, including: regulating baby's heart rate, breathing and temperature; encouraging their natural urge to feed, whether breast or bottle fed; promoting bonding between parents and their new baby; and, for a mother, encouraging the release of hormones relating to breast milk supply and breastfeeding.

5. Newborn needs

A newborn baby has no control over their cry – they have needs, not wants, and this is their way of communicating with you. As this book progresses we will talk about avoiding feeding and rocking to sleep in the long term, but this does not relate to the newborn stage. When your baby is very young they may need help in the form of rocking, swaying, sucking or feeding to regulate their emotions in order to relax enough to be able to fall asleep.

6. Babies are noisy sleepers!

I'm always surprised at how noisy some babies are when they're sleeping or trying to get to sleep. Do not worry. Some new parents tend to pick baby up and rock them because they think something is wrong, but this can be quite normal and the squirming may be part of their digestive process, helping to release trapped wind from both ends. Picking baby up may even wake them. However, if they start to actually cry and sound distressed this is often a sign of wind, so pick them up and put them over your shoulder for a minute.

7. Focus on feeding

In the early days and weeks feeding should be your prime focus. Don't worry about your baby's sleep patterns as this will happen naturally if feeding is good. If your baby has a full tummy and has been winded, they should be content and a good rhythm should begin to fall into place. Although do be aware that a newborn baby's stomach is very tiny, about the size of a cherry at 1 day old, a walnut at 3 days and an apricot at 1 week old.

Make every feed count

Make this your mantra! Whether you are breast- or bottle-feeding, this is so important. If you aim for your baby to get a nice full tummy at each and every feed, they should be satisfied and ready for a good long nap. If you are breastfeeding, encourage your baby to 'actively feed' with a good, deep latch. If your baby is spending a lot of time at the breast, this doesn't necessarily mean they are getting a lot of milk. If the latch is good you should see the lower jaw moving up and down rhythmically, hear swallowing and observe your baby taking small rests. A good latch promotes high milk flow and minimises discomfort, while a poor latch can result in low milk transfer and lead to damaged nipples. If you are unsure of your latch, your midwife, health visitor or a lactation specialist should be able to help.

Encourage 'active' feeding

Active feeding means making sure your baby is actively drinking their milk rather than having a snack and a snooze. If baby falls asleep mid-feed, which they often do as feeding is tiring, stroke their cheeks, tickle their toes or change their nappy to wake them up and feed some more! If they don't wake when you change their nappy, then they have probably had a good full feed.

Wind well during and after a feed, and try to avoid getting into a rhythm of short feeds. For breastfeeding mothers this will also help to prevent baby spending all day on the breast, feeding half-heartedly, thus making your nipples sore and you exhausted.

As a maternity nurse I support parents to establish good feeding patterns from day one. Babies are much easier to settle to sleep in their crib when they have a nice full tummy and this means the parent or carer can rest between feeds. This is the key to good long-term sleep patterns and I'm sure this is why I was successful when breastfeeding my triplets. It also results in the baby feeling comfortable and safe in their sleeping space from the start.

Breastfeeding is not always easy to establish so do please seek support and help if feeding is not going to plan. The earlier you can get help, the better.

Many new parents are unprepared for how exhausting parenthood is in the early months. A newborn baby will need to feed at least every 3 hours and sometimes more while establishing feeding. A feed can take some time, particularly when your baby is newborn, and once you've dealt with your baby's other needs, settled them back to sleep and got yourself back to sleep, it is soon time to feed again! I apologise for the reality check, but this is 24 hours a day, 7 days a week and I think it's important to be prepared for this, so accept any offers of help to give you the opportunity to recharge your batteries and try to take a power nap whenever you can. Thankfully, this tiring phase has the reward of being a most magical time as you get to know your new baby.

Make every feed count.

Part Two:
SLEEP –
THE BASICS

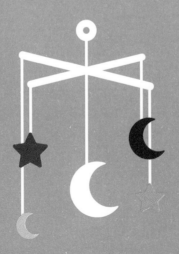

8. Safe sleep

Babies need a lot of sleep during the first few months of their lives so it's important to ensure that they are sleeping as safely as possible.

Sudden infant death syndrome (SIDS) is the sudden and unexplained death of a baby where no cause is found. While SIDS is rare, it can still happen and there are steps that parents can take to help reduce the chance of this tragedy occurring.

The Lullaby Trust, a British charitable organisation, is the recognised national authority on safe sleeping practices for infants and children. It recommends the following advice (for all sleep periods, not just night-time) to significantly reduce the risk of SIDS.

★ **Place your baby to sleep in a separate cot or Moses basket in the same room as you for the first 6 months.**
★ **Always place your baby on their back to sleep, with their feet at the foot of the cot ('feet to foot' position), so that they cannot wriggle under covers. Once they start to roll from front to back by themselves, you can leave them to find their own position for sleep.**
★ **Ensure their sleep space is kept clear of all items and there is nothing within reach of the space, such as window blind cords, nappy sacks or soft toys.**

- ★ Use a firm, flat, mattress in good condition, protected by a waterproof cover.
- ★ Use firmly tucked-in sheets or blankets (not above shoulder height) or a baby sleep bag.
- ★ Do not use pillows, quilts, duvets or bumpers.
- ★ Do not use pods, nests or sleep positioners.
- ★ Make sure your baby's head is kept uncovered.
- ★ Try to keep the room temperature between 16 and 20 degrees Celsius so your baby does not get too hot or cold.
- ★ Make sure bedding is appropriate for the time of year.
- ★ Babies should not be allowed to sleep in bouncy chairs or be left sleeping in the car seat when not travelling in the car.
- ★ Keep your baby's environment smoke-free during pregnancy and after birth.
- ★ Breastfeed your baby, if possible.
- ★ Do not sleep in the same bed as your baby if you or anyone in the same bed as you is extremely tired, has recently drunk alcohol or taken drugs, or if your baby was born prematurely or was of low birth weight.
- ★ If you choose to bed share (see page 22), seek advice on how to do that as safely as possible.
- ★ Never sleep on a sofa or in an armchair with your baby. This can be extremely dangerous for babies.

More information can be found at www.lullabytrust.org.uk.

9. Medical conditions

There are a lot of books on medical conditions, so I will keep this section brief. The most likely problems you may face with an otherwise-healthy baby are colic, reflux, silent reflux or cow's milk protein allergy (CMPA) or intolerance. These can be difficult to diagnose, but if your baby is terribly unhappy day in, day out, is very difficult to settle and seems to be crying in pain, seek medical help. Trust your instincts.

Your baby will be difficult to settle if they experience any of the above so you will need to do a lot more cuddling, rocking and soothing. If you are following medical advice, you may also be advised to feed your baby little and often. In any of these situations, just give your baby the attention they need. I know it's terribly hard and you will be exhausted, but your baby's condition will improve with time and help. Try to sleep when your baby sleeps and accept any offers of assistance. Above all, try not to cope alone.

Babies who experience colic usually start to improve around 3 months old, while with severe reflux, unfortunately, it can take longer. I suggest you do whatever you can to help your baby to settle, but as soon as they are ready and the situation begins to improve, encourage them to self-settle using the gradual retreat process, explained in section 27. Sleep is a great healer.

10. Why is sleep important?

Sleep is essential for the physical and psychological health of your child. Studies have proved that a good night's sleep and regular bedtime routine have a significantly positive impact on a child's well-being, particularly their behaviour and ability to learn. Lack of sleep has been linked with obesity, aggression, behaviour problems, low IQ and poor memory.

Sleep deprivation has a negative impact on the whole family. Sleep-deprived parents are likely to find parenting challenging, and a lack of sleep can have much wider-ranging consequences including a negative effect on parents' relationships with each other and their children.

Sleep problems can be common and are often preventable. Although I will stress the importance of establishing positive sleep habits early on, it's never too late to help your child. Furthermore, studies have shown that children who have good sleep habits are less likely to experience sleep problems such as insomnia in adult life. When you help your child to sleep well, you often see a dramatic improvement in their mood, appetite and behaviour.

A good night's sleep can have a significant impact on a child's health, well-being, behaviour and ability to learn.

> *We embarked on a programme of 'sleep teaching' when my son was 13 months old. Up until then, we had both had very little sleep. It wasn't easy as I had fallen into habits that had to be undone. However, after a couple of months, my son's nursery teacher said that she couldn't believe the change in him, he was so much more content and his appetite had improved.*

Anna, mother of Thomas, aged 16 months

Average sleep needs chart

This chart shows the 'average' sleep needs of a baby or child, but please bear in mind the 'average' can vary greatly between babies, so only refer to this as a guide. The hours of night-time sleep do not necessarily indicate continuous unbroken sleep.

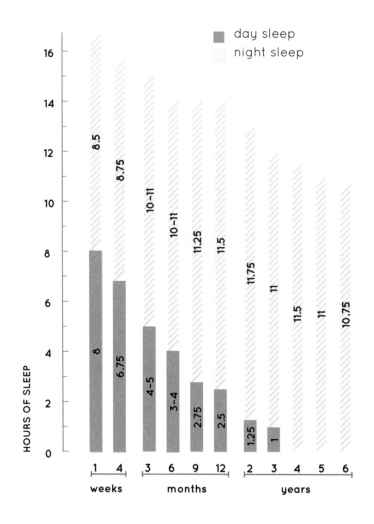

HOURS OF SLEEP

day sleep
night sleep

1	4	weeks
3	6	9	12	months
2	3	4	5	6	years

night sleep values: 8.5, 8.75, 10–11, 10–11, 11.25, 11.5, 11.75, 11, 11.5, 11, 10.75

day sleep values: 8, 6.75, 4–5, 3–4, 2.75, 2.5, 1.25, 1

11. Understanding sleep

Types of sleep

When we go to sleep it's not a simple matter of switching off and waking up in the morning, we go through cycles, experiencing various stages along the way from drowsiness to light sleep, through to deep sleep. Even though your body is resting and restoring its energy levels, sleep is an active state, essential for your physical and mental well-being. We can divide sleep into two broad types:

Non-REM sleep (non-rapid eye movement sleep)

Non-REM sleep is a deep sleep where the brain rests; blood is released to the muscles; tissue is grown or repaired; hormones are released for growth and development; and white blood cells are made to support the immune system. During non-REM sleep your baby will breathe steadily and deeply, and will be hard to wake.

> **Non-REM sleep is not fully developed until your baby is around 4 months old.**

REM sleep (rapid eye movement sleep)

REM sleep is vital to the development of the brain and it is the state in which we dream. The body rests, extra blood is released to the brain and the baby processes what they have seen and heard during the day. Young babies spend a lot of time in REM sleep due to its developmental importance.

> **REM sleep is sometimes known as 'dream sleep'.**

Helping our babies and children to sleep through the night will enable them to achieve a sufficient amount of both types of sleep to aid their development.

Sleep hormones

There are two key hormones connected with sleep and it helps to understand the importance of each.

Melatonin

Also known as the sleep hormone, melatonin regulates sleep by telling your body it's night-time and it's time to go to bed. When your baby goes to sleep at night, it's beneficial for melatonin levels to be high. You can help to influence this by having a good predictable bed- and bath-time routine. Melatonin is produced primarily in darkness, so keep the lights low and avoid any exposure to TV or computer screens close to bedtime as the blue light emitted from such devices inhibits the production of melatonin. A baby's melatonin levels increase around the age of 3 months, so this is your real window of opportunity to establish a routine and encourage positive sleep habits. However, if you miss this window, don't feel disheartened as it is never too late to establish a routine.

> **Keep the lights low at bedtime and avoid exposure to any devices that emit blue light.**

Cortisol

This is the hormone created when the body is overtired and sleep deprived. It's sometimes known as the stress hormone. If your baby's cortisol levels are high, they will find it very difficult to go to sleep, which is why it's important to encourage good daytime naps. Too much cortisol can also cause regular night-time waking and early rising.

You can often see the effect of cortisol in older children who are not good sleepers, they appear to be active, 'wired' and on the go all the time. Parents may think they have a child who needs less sleep than their peers as they are full of energy, but actually their body is releasing cortisol as a way to cope with their fatigue. This is not healthy for the child – they need more sleep.

> **Too much cortisol is like a dose of caffeine!**

12. Sleep cycles

A healthy newborn baby will sleep until one of the following things happen: hunger; discomfort, such as wind or a wet or dirty nappy; or sleep is no longer needed. However, by the age of around 3–4 months your baby's sleep matures and they will start to sleep in cycles progressing through the different stages of sleep – from light sleep to deep sleep. At night, these cycles usually last 60–90 minutes and are marked by a brief waking or arousal at the end of the cycle.

Given the fact that sleep cycles extend and melatonin levels increase from around 3 months of age, your baby should be able to sleep for more extended periods at night by this time.

In addition, the circadian rhythm (better known as the body clock) is maturing at this age. This is the 24-hour sequence of biological cycles that influence patterns of sleeping, waking, rest, hunger, activity, body temperature and hormones. This is why babies and children respond so well to routine to keep these rhythms in harmony.

This is the ideal time to guide your baby into a healthy routine, establish regular feed times, nap times, follow a predictable bath and bedtime routine and encourage self-settling.

Sleep cycle chart

This is a diagram to illustrate how a typical 6-month-plus baby goes through a roller-coaster of sleep cycles throughout the night, transitioning through various stages of sleep, from drowsiness to light sleep, through to deep (non-REM) sleep and experiencing periods of dream (REM) sleep along the way. These are also known as sleep stages 1–3.

The periods of brief waking throughout the night are nature's way of checking that our environment is safe. These brief wakings can become a problem if a baby or child cannot settle themselves back to sleep alone and require the help of a parent or a feed to get themselves back to sleep again.

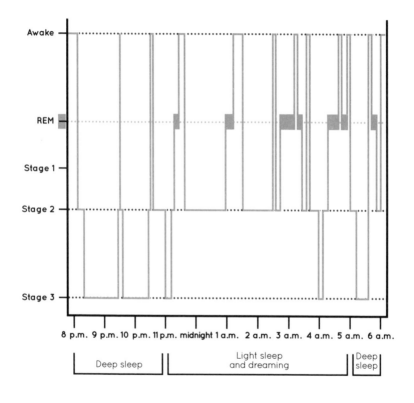

13. Understanding sleep cycles will help you to help your baby

From 3–4 months of age your baby will be rousing approximately every 60–90 minutes during the night. This is possibly the most important fact about your baby's sleep that you need to grasp. It is normal for babies to wake regularly during the night, this is nature's way of keeping us safe, but the key to prevent them from fully waking is for them to have the ability to settle themselves back to sleep again. Alongside the ability to self-settle your baby needs to find themself in exactly the same conditions when they rouse as when they fell asleep at the start of the night. Having the security that 'all is well' will give them the confidence to drift off again and only fully wake if they are hungry or have other needs.

Here are some examples of scenarios to explain the importance of helping your baby to feel safe and secure:

Your baby falls asleep in your arms, being cuddled or rocked. You move them to their cot while they are asleep. During the night they rouse – and instead of finding themself in the warm arms of a parent they are alone in their cot. They do not understand how they have got there, and therefore wake and cry so they can be rocked or cuddled to sleep again. This is the equivalent to you falling asleep in your bed and waking up on the floor!

Your baby nurses to sleep or falls asleep while sucking on their bottle and then you put them in their cot. During the night, they rouse. They are unable to get back to sleep independently as they only know how to get to sleep while sucking. They therefore need to be nursed or fed back to sleep. It can be hard to break the cycle once this is an established habit.

Your baby falls asleep in their cot with the musical mobile playing. There is noise and movement, maybe even a light show. When they rouse during the night it's silent and still. They are disturbed by the change in their conditions and therefore cry for attention.

Your baby is put into their cot drowsy but awake. They fall asleep unaided in their cot, with no music or props. They may have a little cry. This is absolutely normal. It's rarely a cry of distress; your baby is helping themself to get off to sleep. I think of this as letting off steam or releasing tension. When they rouse between sleep cycles during the night, they find themself in exactly the same conditions that they fell asleep in. They feel safe and secure, and they connect to their next sleep cycle unaided. They may have a moan, grizzle or cry while doing this, which is quite normal. Don't be tempted to lift them unless they are distressed or due a feed.

> **It is normal for babies to wake regularly during the night – this is nature's way of keeping them safe.**

Part Three:
ESTABLISHING POSITIVE SLEEP HABITS

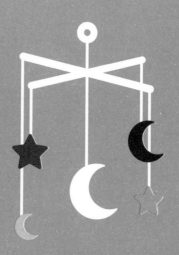

14. Teach the difference between night and day

A newborn baby does not know the difference between night and day, they are simply governed by hunger. In fact, newborns are often on an opposite rhythm to you because, while in the womb, they are rocked and soothed to sleep all day with your movement and voice, and at night, while you are lying still, they wake. It can take a little time to reverse that pattern.

However, from as early as a couple of weeks old, you can help your baby to learn to distinguish night from day by doing the following:

During the day
- ★ Make sure you interact and play with your baby frequently throughout the day.
- ★ Ensure your baby is exposed to plenty of fresh air and daylight by going out for walks or just being out in the garden or the park.
- ★ Don't minimise noise around the house. Carry on as normal so your baby gets used to everyday sounds, like the radio, vacuum cleaner, telephone, etc.
- ★ Draw the curtains when they nap, but don't feel the need to use blackout blinds.

★ During the first month, don't let them sleep for longer than 3–4 hours without a feed. Gently guide them into taking more calories during the daytime.

During the night

★ Have a predictable bedtime routine with sleep cues.
★ Keep lights low while preparing for bedtime as bright lights suppress the production of melatonin, the sleep hormone.
★ Change them into night-time clothing or use a baby sleeping bag.
★ Draw curtains and use blackout blinds if you have them.
★ Make sure their room is warm and cosy, but not too hot, and check for draughts.
★ Keep night feeds focused, have the lights as low as possible and stay in the bedroom.
★ Do not play or chat with your baby, just whisper and keep interaction to a minimum.

You need to be a very different person when you tend to your baby in the night compared to during the day. Be boring! Avoid interaction and keep your voice low. In the morning throw open the curtains, smile and totally engage using your happy daytime voice.

> **Be boring during the night!**

15. Sleep associations

A newborn baby may need lots of help to settle. You will need to comfort them to regulate their emotions enough to help them relax sufficiently in order to fall asleep. Feeding and rocking to sleep may be necessary at this newborn stage, but as babies develop they can learn to fall asleep in response to alternative external cues from their carer.

Every baby is unique and has different temperaments, but helping them learn to self-settle at a young age is usually the best time to start. By establishing positive sleep habits early on, you should hopefully set up a sleeping routine that benefits both parent or carer and child and helps to avoid sleep problems later on.

Helping your baby to discover their own way of self-settling is a fundamental step in encouraging them to sleep through the night. If your baby has fallen asleep dependent on any kind of prop, they may wake repeatedly during the night and need to be helped back to sleep again. Parents often tell me that their baby will only go to sleep while being rocked or fed. These are the sleep cues that their baby has come to associate with sleep so they need to teach their baby to self-settle with alternative cues and thereby develop strategies to help them connect their sleep cycles independently during the night.

A short-term fix can easily
become a long-term habit.

Common sleep associations or 'props'

* Feeding to sleep – breast or bottle
* Rocking
* Cuddling
* Bouncing on an exercise ball
* Sucking on a carer's finger
* Patting
* Music
* Motion – car/pushchair
* Dummy

Try to establish positive sleep habits early on.

Dummies

Whether or not you should use a dummy as a pacifier for your baby is a matter of constant debate. There seems to be little concrete evidence to suggest the benefit or harm in the long term, however, the Lullaby Trust's guidelines state that some research suggests it is possible that using a dummy when putting a baby down to sleep might reduce the risk of sudden infant death syndrome. It advises not to give a dummy to a baby before the age of 4 weeks and – if you are breastfeeding – to wait until breastfeeding is well established, usually around 4–6 weeks, before introducing a dummy. This should avoid your baby getting 'nipple confusion', which is the term used when a baby has difficulty latching onto the breast due to the early introduction of a dummy or a teat, which involves using a different sucking technique. Additionally, dummies can also mask hunger in newborn babies. The Lullaby Trust advises to then stop using the dummy when your baby is 6–12 months old. However, in my opinion it can be quite difficult to remove a dummy at this stage as your baby will have learnt to go to sleep sucking so it will be a strong sleep association.

If a baby has learnt to fall asleep sucking a dummy this is likely to be the only way they can easily fall asleep. This can become a problem as, inevitably, the dummy parts company with baby during a sleep cycle and when baby needs to suck on the dummy to connect to the next sleep cycle they are not physically able to find it and put it back into their mouth. Baby then cries and their parent or carer has to come and pop the dummy back in. This can happen repeatedly during the night, so it's something to be aware of if you choose to use one. To help an older baby to find their dummy during the night you can purchase small soft toys that the dummies easily attach to and these make it easier for baby to locate it independently in the night.

Ideally you will teach your baby to sleep without the aid of a prop, but at the end of the day you are the only person who can judge what is right for your baby in your circumstances. Premature babies are often given dummies in hospital to help stimulate their suck before they are able to breast- or bottle-feed efficiently, and if you have a baby suffering from colic or reflux, sucking on a dummy can be a great source of comfort to them; just try not to use the dummy continually and give it only when necessary.

Breastfeeding as a sleep aid

In the early weeks nursing for comfort is positively encouraged to help your baby get used to this world, but in the longer term they may become dependent on nursing as a sleep aid – which can be a difficult habit to break. If this is your long-term choice and its working for you, there is no need to make any changes, however, if you would like your baby to have a little sleep independence, consider the following.

Has your baby finished breastfeeding? Gently unlatch your baby from the breast, wind them and then have some play and interaction time.

When you are giving your baby their last feed before bedtime, try not to allow them to fall asleep on the breast. It's unavoidable when they are tiny, but from around the age of 10–16 weeks, wind them, have a cuddle and try to put them down drowsy but awake enough to be aware of their surroundings. Once your baby is old enough to take an interest in books, enjoy a short story together before settling them into their cot, to disassociate feeding and sleeping. If they are difficult to settle, see section 22.

Try to use the breast as a food supply rather than teaching your baby to become dependent on it as a source of comfort. If your baby uses the breast as a sleep aid, they will not be able to go to sleep in any other way, and as they get older your baby may wake regularly between every sleep cycle at night and need you to feed them back to sleep again.

The exception to this is during the early weeks when you are bonding and establishing milk supply.

> **Breastfeeding to sleep can be
> a difficult habit to break.**

" *I met up with Stephanie when my baby was 6 months old. As we were talking he started to grizzle and root for milk. Stephanie asked me if he was hungry, I said that he shouldn't be as he had fed recently. She suggested that I put him to the breast so that she could observe and he immediately started to fall asleep. He was using me as a dummy! That's when I changed my routine. I had been finding breastfeeding exhausting as he wanted to be at the breast much of the time and I was considering stopping altogether, but once I weaned him off feeding for comfort and started to just use the breast for food, we were both much happier!*

Marilyn, mother of Lucas, aged 6 months

Create a positive sleep association

Encourage your baby to form an attachment to some sort of comforter. This could be a safe, small soft toy or a small soft cloth square with silky labels attached – you'll work out what is favoured by your baby and, inevitably, it will end up having a name such as a 'lovey'. Make sure the item is safe – do not put a large blanket in their cot that they could cover their face with. It's essential to have duplicates so that you can switch them for a wash.

You are aiming for this comforter to become a sleep 'trigger', so each time you place it with your baby they may caress it, rub it between their fingers and become soporific. This is what your baby will turn to for comfort in the middle of the night when they wake briefly between sleep cycles and it will help them to self-soothe. Current SIDS guidelines advise that you should not place soft toys or anything that could cover your baby's face or head in the cot in the first 12 months. However, you can familiarise your baby with the comforter before then, keeping it against your skin to give it a comforting, reassuring smell, and then give it to your baby to hold when you are having a cuddle. Once they are old enough to have their comforter at sleep times, place it in their hand as you lay them in their cot. Not all babies form an attachment with a comforter, but when they do it can become a strong and positive sleep association that is portable, always giving your baby a feeling of comfort and security.

> **Encourage a loving attachment with a comforter or 'lovey'. Only give the comforter to your baby at sleep and nap times or it may lose its magic!**

White noise

White noise can be played for nap times and night times. This background noise can calm babies and help them to fall asleep quicker, some emulate the sound of the womb or make shushing sounds. Depending on the frequency of the sound it can also be known as pink or brown noise.

If this is played at every sleep time it can become a sleep association or dependence but it's a positive sleep association as it does not require parental intervention. The most important thing is to keep it on all night or for the whole nap so your baby's conditions don't change mid sleep.

Another advantage of white noise is that it can mask distractive sounds such as traffic, creaking floorboards or snoring parents!

16. Demand feeding

Demand feeding, also known as responsive feeding, means feeding your baby whenever they signal that they are hungry, usually by crying, rooting or sucking on their hands, rather than according to a set schedule.

By all means demand feed your baby, but endeavour to not feed at every demand!

Let me elaborate... In the early days and weeks while you are establishing your milk supply and bonding with your baby you will need to breastfeed little and often. This will help your milk supply, encourage bonding with your baby and help them to learn the technique to take a good feed. Your baby has a tiny tummy and cannot take in large volumes so will have to feed frequently.

Likewise, if you are bottle feeding, feed your baby when they show signs of hunger and let them feed for as long as they want to. In the early days, this will be little and often. You will learn to recognise your baby's hunger cues and their 'hungry' cry.

However, once feeding is established, after the first month or so, start to space your feeds gradually and ensure that every feed is a good, focused feed. If you are feeding every 2 hours, increase to 2.25 hours for a couple of days, then 2.5 hours and so on. Once your baby is able to take bigger feeds, less often, this will help them to sleep for longer periods during the night.

As your baby gets older, if you allow them to constantly 'snack feed' they are unlikely to take enough food to sustain them through naps of a restorative length, and if they have snack feeds during the day they may want to snack feed at regular intervals at night. If you are breastfeeding, your milk gradually increases in fat and calorific content during a feed, so encouraging your baby to take a full feed is likely to satisfy them for longer. For this reason, it is important not to switch breasts while your baby is actively nursing.

Do not meet every emotional need with food

In a world where obesity is on the increase, we must be aware not to meet every need or quell every cry with food. Babies cry for all manner of reasons – they're wet, they're tired, they're in pain, they're bored – so it's important to establish why your baby is crying and what they need. If you always meet their cry with a breast to nurse on or a bottle of milk to keep them quiet, then they may grow up feeling that food is the answer to every emotional need.

> **Assess your baby's needs; don't just assume they are hungry.**

17. Let your baby have a voice

Crying is your baby's only form of communication. Pause, observe and listen. If you immediately quell every cry, how can you understand what your baby is trying to tell you?

* **Are they hungry?**
* **Are they bored?**
* **Are they uncomfortable?**
* **Do they have wind?**
* **Do they need a nappy change?**
* **Are they too hot/too cold?**
* **Are they unwell?**
* **Are they trying to connect sleep cycles? This may often involve a little crying or grizzling.**

Try to differentiate between their cries. Babies have different cries for different needs. Are they actually crying because they are distressed and hungry, or are they letting off some steam and trying to settle themself to sleep?

> *One of the most valuable things you have taught me is simply to 'allow my baby her voice'. Before you said that to me, I was always desperate to find the quickest way to stop her from crying. Now I understand that sometimes she just needs to cry and I've learnt to differentiate her cries much better.*
>
> Toni, mother of Willow, aged 5 months

18. The pause

I think 'pausing' is a very important part of understanding your baby. Don't react to them too quickly; pause, observe and listen. If your baby is ever going to learn to connect their sleep cycles independently you have to give them the opportunity to do so! If you pick them up the moment they cry, you may even be waking them.

I am not saying let your baby wail or cry in distress – absolutely not – just listen, assess and don't rush in as soon as they stir. Babies can be very noisy when learning how to connect sleep cycles; it may involve some crying, moaning or grumbling.

Babies are often noisy sleepers and, because current guidelines recommend that your baby sleeps in your room until 6 months of age, it is very easy for a parent to react too quickly to their baby's cry because they don't want their partner to be disturbed. This is understandable if one parent has an early start and a long day of work ahead, but these quick reactions can actually wake the baby when, if they were left for a few minutes, they may have self-settled. Rushing to your baby's every stir or grizzle means you are basically connecting their sleep cycles for them, never allowing them the opportunity to learn to self-settle, which will subsequently encourage regular waking. If their grizzle becomes a cry of need, you then, of course, attend to them. Allowing a pause will help in the long term. If one of the parents is working with machinery or doing a lot of driving, you may wish to consider sleeping in separate bedrooms for the first few weeks.

Parents of second and subsequent children often say that their babies are more contented and better sleepers than the first. This is usually because the carer is busier and more distracted, and therefore gives the second child the opportunity to learn to self-settle and connect their own sleep cycles.

> **Give your baby the opportunity to learn to connect their sleep cycles independently.**

"" *I do feel that putting into practice the lessons you taught me has helped already, even though Olivia is only 4 weeks old. You have given me the confidence to take a step back and pause to see exactly why she is stirring and whether she is just trying to get herself to sleep, which she actually often does.* ""

Serena, mother of Olivia, aged 4 weeks

19. Feeding at night

When you feed your baby during the night, you do not need to wake them before putting them back down to sleep (this is only essential at the start of the night). Give the feed, either breast or bottle, keeping interaction to a minimum, then wind your baby and settle them back into the cot as quickly as possible. Only change the nappy during the night if absolutely necessary.

As your baby gets older, don't always assume they need a night feed when they wake. If they have had a good feed 2 hours previously, they shouldn't need feeding again. Simply resettle them. It may be difficult at first, but with consistency it will get easier because your baby will soon learn that you are not going to feed them every 2 hours during the night.

As a new parent it can be difficult to know how often to feed. In the early weeks, if you are 'demand' feeding (see page 59), your baby may feed little and often. However, if you are feeding every 3 hours during the day and they are waking hourly at night, a feed is probably not the answer and your baby may just need some comfort and help to resettle.

Bottle-fed babies can often settle into a more structured routine early on, but with a breastfed baby it can be more difficult as you cannot be certain of how much milk your baby has taken at a particular feed. It can really help to keep a diary of feeds, and if your baby is feeding every 3 or 4 hours in the day, they should not need to feed more often than that at night. If they are settling independently at the start of the night they should sleep for longer and longer stretches during the night, naturally dropping night feeds and only rousing between sleep cycles if they are genuinely hungry.

> **If your baby wakes in the night, don't always assume they need a feed – they may just need some help resettling.**

Dream feeds

Many parenting advisors recommend 'dream feeding' your baby at around 10 or 11 p.m. before the parents go to bed. As the name suggests, this involves feeding your baby while they are still asleep. The theory is that by doing this the parents 'hopefully' get to have a longer stretch of uninterrupted sleep when they themselves are in their deep sleep phase.

I have mixed feelings about this. I feel that by dream feeding you are interrupting your baby's natural rhythms, disturbing their sleep pattern development and are feeding them when they are not hungry. Moreover, at around 10 or 11 p.m., your baby is in their deep non-REM sleep phase, a time of important physical development, so I do not feel you should stimulate the digestive system when it wants to rest.

By dream feeding you're in danger of creating a learnt hunger in your baby at that time. Whereas if you allow your baby's natural rhythms to develop, the length of time they sleep should gradually increase, especially during this period of deep sleep when they should find it easier to connect their sleep cycles.

In my mind, a much better solution is for the parents to have an early night so that they can achieve a decent period of deep sleep before being woken. Remember, this difficult period of adjusting to your baby's sleep patterns is such a short time in the grand scheme of things, that a little compromise on your part as a parent can really pay dividends in the long term.

How to wean your baby off night feeds

At around 6 months old, your baby should no longer need regular night feeds, provided they are feeding well in the day and are in good health. Feeding during the night stimulates their metabolism at a time when they should be resting. If you have helped them to self-settle from a young age they may well have stopped waking for feeds long ago. If they are still waking this may be a learnt habit that can be changed.

Regular night feeding also creates a negative cycle where your baby is filling up on calories during the night so is not needing to eat so much in the day. Once you wean off night feeds, you should see their appetite improve during the day. If you have a particularly hungry baby, your baby has medical issues or if you have any doubts, consult your GP or health visitor before reducing night feeds.

If your baby has learnt to self-settle at the start of the night you can gently and gradually eliminate night feeds. If your baby is still feeding to sleep at the start of the night you need to address this issue before attempting to cut out night feeds. See sections 22 and 27.

There are two techniques to reduce night feeding. The first is to decrease the amount of milk you are giving your baby at each feed. For a bottle-fed baby, gradually reduce the volume of milk given over a period of nights. For example, you can reduce the volume by 15–30 ml (½–1 fl oz), each night until you reach 60 ml (2 fl oz) and then stop altogether and use a settling technique to help your baby get back to sleep. For a breastfed baby, gradually reduce the number of minutes offered at the breast over a period of nights and, once you are down to a couple of minutes, stop altogether and use a settling technique.

The second technique is to increase the interval between feeds. For example, if your baby is feeding every 3 hours, increase the time between feeds to 3.5 hours for two nights, then 4 hours for two nights and so on.

Choose one method or the other, you do not need to do both. Your baby should gradually wake less for milk and eventually give it up altogether; if not, you will need to implement a settling technique to help them get back to sleep. However, your baby should have gradually adjusted to eating less during the night so is less likely to experience hunger and their appetite should improve during the day.

As I have said before, it's crucial that you are consistent. Once you have stopped night feeding, try not to go back to it. This will confuse your baby. If they wake during the night because, for example, they are teething or unwell, give them love, comfort, cuddles, water – if necessary for a baby over 6 months old – and any medication that a health professional has recommended. If you are tempted to feed your baby to get them back to sleep, you may disrupt all the good work you have done to wean them off night feeds and this will affect their appetite during the day, once again creating a negative cycle and confusion.

Also, do not be lured into feeding your baby to keep them quiet in other tricky situations, such as when you are on holiday and their sleep patterns have been slightly disrupted, or when you're staying with friends and you feel awkward about them potentially waking the household. It may seem like the easy option at the time, but it is unfair on your baby and will cause confusion.

> **The golden rules are time, repetition and consistency.**

20. Routine

Babies love routine! I don't believe in a rigid feeding and sleeping routine, I think there needs to be some flexibility, but I do think that babies who have a routine are often more content and so are their parents. Instead of clock watching, try to think of it as a sequence of events with a consistent pattern and work at your baby's pace.

Once your baby is around 6-8 weeks old try to establish a regular daytime feed and nap routine to avoid your baby becoming overtired. Learn your baby's rhythms and establish a routine tailored to your lifestyle and situation.

Keep a note of when your baby sleeps and for how long; this will help you to understand your baby's rhythm. If you keep nap times regular your baby will get used to sleeping at that time and they will find it easier to fall asleep.

This is not an exact science. All babies differ, but here are some guidelines:

6–12 weeks – A nap every 1–2 hours.

3–6 months – A nap every 2–3 hours.

6–9 months – Three naps, gradually reducing to two. In the morning, one sleep cycle (approximately 45–60 minutes). Lunch time, at least two sleep cycles (approximately 90 minutes plus). Afternoon, one sleep cycle or catnap, depending on age and length of the lunchtime nap. Babies are often difficult to settle for this afternoon nap, so this could be a nap triggered by you taking them for a stroll in the pushchair or a baby carrier/sling. The third nap is usually dropped between 6–8 months. Reduce the length of this nap slowly until it's no longer needed.

9–12 months – Two naps. Morning, one sleep cycle. Post lunch, at least two sleep cycles.

12 months plus – You can now work towards one nap a day. Some babies will do this earlier than others, but when you feel they are ready (usually between 14–18 months), you may need to bring lunchtime forward to 11.30 a.m. for a transitional period and then put baby down for a long nap straight after, aiming at 2 hours. Once your baby has adjusted to this new routine you can gradually move lunch back to your usual time.

2–3 years – Your child will probably have one lunchtime nap of 1–1.5 hours at this time, shortening as they get nearer to 3 years, although some will completely drop their nap before the age of three. However, you need to try to avoid your child becoming so overtired that he drops off late afternoon, as a late sleep will affect bedtime.

3 years plus – Although a nap isn't usually necessary at this age, I think it's good to encourage a quiet period after lunch, maybe reading stories or listening to audio books.

Learn your baby's rhythms.

"
*Once I got my twins into
a manageable routine, I began
to enjoy them so much more,
they became happier, generally
more contented and I got a
little time to myself too!*
"

Rachel, mother of Toby and Zoe, aged 8 months

Feeding and napping routine

Once you have passed the sleepy newborn stage, establish a routine that does not involve feeding just before napping. This is key! To avoid developing a feed-to-sleep association I would recommend feeding your baby shortly after they have woken from their nap rather than just before they go back down for their next nap. This has the added advantage that it should encourage your baby to take a good, full feed as they won't be falling asleep while feeding. A positive sleep/awake pattern to follow is:

Nap
Feed
Play/interaction
Nap

If you do need to feed just before your baby is due a nap, try not to feed them to sleep. If your baby is dropping off, tickle their feet, wind them and maybe have a look at a picture book or sing a lullaby to break the association between feeding and sleeping, and then put baby in their cot or Moses basket, drowsy but awake. If your older baby is hungry at nap time try giving them milk from a beaker to avoid them sucking to sleep.

Once feeding is well established or by at least 2 months old, try to elongate the time between feeds. If your baby is taking good full feeds this should happen naturally, but if you are feeding every 2 hours, gradually move on to every 3 hours by increasing the interval between feeds by 15 minutes every couple of days until you reach the desired time between feeds. If your baby feeds every 2 hours or less they will only be able to take a small feed each time – which will not sustain them through their next nap – but by gradually extending this time they will be able to take a bigger and more satisfying feed. This will help them to sleep longer at night too. If you feel they are ready, you can move on to feeding them every 4 hours. Some babies never move onto 4-hourly feeding, it very much depends on the baby and the volume of milk they like to take. Do what works best for you and your baby.

> *Having fallen into the trap of nursing my first baby to sleep, I found it really difficult to settle her in any other way and I didn't want to do the same again. Therefore, with my second daughter, I chose a pattern of feeding shortly after waking rather than just before a nap. This was so much easier as my daughter didn't associate feeding with sleeping. Quite early on, I also worked towards establishing an organised but flexible feeding and napping schedule. This helped me to fit in with my older daughter's activities and my baby was generally more contented and a much better sleeper than my first.*

Amelia, mother of Sophia, aged 3,
and Maisie, aged 9 months

Bath/bed routine

If you haven't established a bath and bedtime routine by the time your baby is 3 months old, then this is the ideal time to implement it.

A regular and predictable bath routine is essential. It relaxes your baby and helps melatonin levels to rise. This is the sleep hormone discussed in section 11, which will help your baby settle more easily. A routine also creates cues to help your baby to understand the difference between night-time and daytime sleep. Babies learn by association, so quickly get used to a repetitive pattern.

★ **Your routine should commence at the same time every night and take no longer than 30–45 minutes. If you make your routine longer than this, your baby will lose focus and you will not benefit from the melatonin rise.**

★ **Plan your routine around a time that fits in with your family life and other children. For example, there is no point in bathing your baby, having them all warm, cosy and drowsy, and then your partner comes home and wants to play. You will lose all the advantages you have gained, and your baby will probably go to bed overtired and overstimulated.**

★ **Avoid exposing your baby to TV or computer screens in the early evening as the blue light from such devices inhibits the production of melatonin.**

★ **Around 7 p.m. for bedtime, or a little earlier, seems to fit in with many families, so that would mean commencing your routine around 6.15–6.30 p.m., but having quiet time before then. In countries with a very hot climate a later bedtime often works better, once the temperature has dropped.**

From around 4 months of age, it's best to give your baby their last feed before their bath. This way, you are completely disassociating feeding and sleeping. This can also be helpful for colicky/windy babies, as it enables the baby to get their wind up before settling to sleep. If you avoid giving a full feed after bath your baby is less likely to fall asleep on the breast or bottle. Once your baby is used to this routine it works very well. However, some parents feel this goes against instinct and worry that bathing with a full stomach will be uncomfortable for their baby, but remember this night-time bath should be short, calming and relaxing, so this really isn't an issue. An alternative, often more favoured compromise is to do a split feed; give half before and half after bath. If you do this, ensure your baby does not fall asleep while feeding and read a story or sing a lullaby between feeding and putting into the cot to create a gap between food and sleep.

Give your baby a warm, soothing and quiet, short bath, rather than a playful experience. After the bath, wrap baby in a towel, and give them a massage if you like, then dress them in night clothes and take them into the bedroom. When you take your baby out of their warm bath, they experience a temperature drop and this creates a boost of melatonin. Do not go back to the living area, as this will stimulate your baby. Have the lights low in the bedroom and quietly look at a book or sing a lullaby together. Your routine can be whatever you want it to be as long as it's quiet and gentle. The most important thing is that you do the same every night. Make it predictable so baby understands it is bedtime.

Remember, we are aiming for drowsy but awake! If you play soothing music during your routine, turn it off now and place your baby in their cot, say soothing words and explain that it's sleep time. Soothe if necessary, but for your baby to sleep through the night they need to learn to fall asleep independently, without your presence.

Remember to ensure that the conditions they fall asleep in are the conditions they will find themself in when they rouse during the night. For example, don't play music: when they rouse, it will be silent. Don't leave a light on and then turn it off later: when they rouse, it will be dark. A low plug-in night light is ideal so you can see if you need to attend to them.

Put your baby into their cot drowsy but awake.

> *My baby often cries himself to sleep but it's a grizzle rather than a cry of distress. I give him 5 minutes or so and if he hasn't settled I check on him in case he has a bit of wind or a dirty nappy.*

Sarah, mother of Max, aged 4 months

Sleep cue words

When you put your baby down for a sleep, during the day, night or in the middle of the night, say the same reassuring words from day one. Something like, 'Night night, my darling, it's sleep time now. I love you' and give a kiss and a cuddle. Sleep cue words are powerful and reassuring; get your partner, childminder, nanny, whoever, to use the same words.

21. Naps

Daytime naps are so important. It's a myth that if babies sleep during the day they won't sleep at night – the opposite is true! Sleep encourages sleep. If your baby is well rested they will find it easier to go to sleep at night, will be more content and have a healthier appetite. If you restrict naps, your baby will be overtired, cortisol levels will increase (see section 11 – Sleep hormones), they may find it difficult to get to sleep, and be more prone to night waking and early rising.

The timing of naps will affect your baby's 24-hour cycle. If you're trying to put them down to sleep when they are overtired or under-tired it may be a battle. It's a fine balance, which needs fine tuning for a good night's sleep. To add complications, a baby's nap needs change as they get older.

Create a mini-nap routine with sleep cues. For example, after some gentle quiet play or lullabies, go to where your baby takes their nap, read a short story and settle them into their cot, gently explaining that it's sleep time. Parents quite often have difficulty in getting their babies to nap in their cots during the day and end up taking them for a walk or a drive at every nap time. This is acceptable in the short term for creating a regular sleep pattern, but try to encourage a sleep in the cot or Moses basket at least once a day. If your baby is not keen, be persistent and try every now and again, but don't worry about it, a nap is a nap wherever it may be.

The secret to good napping is getting the spacing between each nap right. This is where a sleep diary is beneficial. It will help you to understand your baby's rhythms. Look for sleep cues, which are sometimes very subtle, and don't wait until your baby is overtired to put them down for a nap.

Sleep cues

- ★ **Staring**
- ★ **Loss of interest in people and toys**
- ★ **Decreased activity**
- ★ **Less vocal**
- ★ **Burying their face into your chest**
- ★ **Rubbing eyes**
- ★ **Pulling ears**
- ★ **Yawning and stretching**
- ★ **Whining and crying**

If you put your baby down for their first nap of the day too early you may encourage early rising, if you put them down too late in the day, you may have problems at bedtime, as your baby will be less likely to be tired.

During the day, it is common for babies to sleep in approximately 30–45-minute sleep cycles so you will probably find that naps are either one or two sleep cycles in length.

Try to encourage fewer but longer naps to help your baby gain the full physiological benefits that deeper sleep offers. Make adjustments gradually – if you try to space naps too rapidly, your baby may become overtired and grumpy. A good rule of thumb is to aim to move on by 15 minutes every couple of days.

Remember, any adjustments you make will take time to kick in. Don't make changes and, after two or three days, think, 'This is not working, I'll change it.' You will end up with a very confused baby.

TIME, REPETITION AND CONSISTENCY are key!

If you find your baby difficult to settle for naps, see section 22.

Sleep encourages sleep!

22. How to settle your baby

The younger your baby, the easier it is to help them to self-settle.

0-2 months – Anything goes! This is a time for bonding and getting to know your baby. They may need a lot of comfort and cuddles in these early weeks along with help to settle and connect their sleep cycles. However, do give them the opportunity to sleep in their cot or Moses basket. Although it's lovely to hold a sleeping baby, they need to feel comfortable in their own space, so giving early opportunities for this will be beneficial in the long term.

2-3 months – Your baby may enjoy sleeping in your arms. This is fine some of the time but isn't practical in the long term, so the most beneficial thing you can do at this age is to help them to fall asleep in their own space. When they are ready for a nap, have a clean nappy and are not hungry, settle them into their cot, say your reassuring sleep words and put a firm comforting hand on them, then step back and leave them to self-settle. They may cry a little; if this crying escalates try to soothe them with some shushing and patting. If the crying continues to escalate, pick them up and comfort them. Once they are calm but before they are asleep lay them down and start the process again. This is what's known as a 'trust technique'. If you continue to do this until they are asleep, you are giving the message: 'I'm here for you, I will respond to you and I will love and comfort you, but I want you to go to sleep in your cot.'

Be positive and confident and try not to rely on one parent or carer always doing the settling so your baby doesn't get too dependent on one particular person.

3-6 months – If you have not helped your baby to self-settle before now you may have to be a little more persistent, but if you are consistent it will pay off. As above, try to settle them in their cot, say your reassuring sleep words and put a comforting firm hand on them.

Walk away, but if your baby's crying escalates to more than a grizzle or sleepy cry go back to them and shush pat and comfort them. The crucial thing is to see it through until sleep is achieved. However much your baby protests, just stay with them, continue to settle them, almost cuddle them in their cot if you have to. Try to resist picking them up, but if you feel you need to once they are calm and before they are asleep lay them back down and start again. You are not abandoning them to their cries and they will not feel unloved a you are staying with them and giving reassurance. D the same at every sleep situation and each time the achieve sleep in this way, however long it takes, it will b easier the next time. If you are consistent with this yo will be amazed how quickly the teaching process is, bu I must stress that you have to see it through.

This is what's known as a 'gradual retreat' process, s once your baby is comfortable to go to sleep with you help and soothing, you need to move to the next degre of separation to avoid them becoming dependent on you presence to get to sleep. Your next step will be to use les intervention, so less patting and soothing, maybe just a occasional pat and shush. The retreat continues until yo are ready to just sit next to their cot if necessary.

If you are teaching this from a young age you will mov through the steps more quickly. Be mindful that your go is to teach your baby to settle without your presence so you are aiming to lay them in their cot after a cuddle, say goodnight and leave the room. For more information on gradual retreat, see section 27 – Techniques to help your baby learn to settle independently.

It is very difficult to put a timescale on how long this process will take. It will depend on how old your baby is and whether you have always cuddled, rocked or fed them to sleep in the past. Some babies will respond more quickly than others, so it could take three or four days or it could take two or three weeks for you to be able to settle them and then leave the room. In some cases, your presence may be over-stimulating, so it might be more beneficial to just leave your baby to self-settle. However, the most important thing is to be consistent and not change tack after a few nights – this will just confuse your baby.

Remember that babies can be noisy when settling. It may involve 5 minutes of crying or grizzling – listen to and learn your baby's cries. They may just be a bit cross, or letting off a bit of steam and tension. This is normal – only intervene if your baby is distressed.

If your baby is just learning how to self-settle it's always easier to start with the night-time as you have the advantage of higher melatonin levels, which induce a feeling of drowsiness. Once you have introduced self-settling at night, then you can move on to nap times. Choose your baby's most predictable nap, the one where they usually settle the easiest. This is generally the morning nap. Avoid the late-afternoon nap as this is often when they find settling more difficult and are more likely to just catnap.

If your baby is struggling to settle, think about the following:

* **Are they hungry?**
* **Are they overtired?**
* **Are they under-tired?**
* **Do they have wind?**
* **Do they have a dirty nappy?**
* **They may have abdominal discomfort and need a bowel movement?**
* **Are they too hot/too cold?**
* **Are they feeling unwell/teething?**

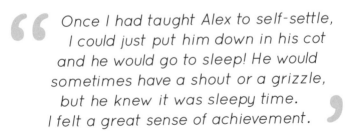

Once I had taught Alex to self-settle, I could just put him down in his cot and he would go to sleep! He would sometimes have a shout or a grizzle, but he knew it was sleepy time. I felt a great sense of achievement.

Jan, mother of Alex, aged 6 months

Swaddling

Swaddling is the technique of snuggly wrapping your baby in a cotton sheet or specially designed swaddling wrap to mirror the sensation of being in the womb. It can give your baby a feeling of security and may help to trigger sleep in the first few weeks. It can also prevent your baby waking themself up with the Moro reflex, also known as the 'startle reflex'. This is an involuntary response which is present for the first 3–6 months.

If you decide to swaddle, it is essential to follow safe-practise guidelines: do not use a blanket or thick fabric as your baby may overheat, and make sure that their face is not covered. You must also ensure that you do not swaddle too tightly around the legs and hips as this can cause hip dysplasia (problems with the hips). Your baby's legs need to be able to move into a natural 'frog-like' position.

I swaddled my triplets and found it to be a very effective sleep cue. From birth, after swaddle-wrapping my babies, I lay them in their Moses baskets and allowed them to self-settle as I simply didn't have the capability to rock three babies at the same time. However, not all babies enjoy being swaddled.

If your baby is premature or has any medical conditions, take advice from your paediatrician on swaddling.

It is advisable to stop swaddling by 10–12 weeks as your baby will become more physically active at this time. Once they start to roll, stop swaddling entirely. They may also want to suck on their thumb or fingers to help them to self-settle.

Monitors

A monitor will allow you to listen to or see your baby when you are in another room. Some also have sensor pads that detect breathing and movement. There is a vast range on the market so you will need to research the options within your budget.

Video monitors are excellent as they allow parents to watch and assess whether intervention is needed. As I've said many times already, babies can be quite noisy and move around quite a lot while connecting their sleep cycles or self-settling. If you are just focusing on listening it can sound quite loud and you may well go in and wake a sleeping baby. Sometimes you will watch a baby crying on the monitor but their eyes are actually closed – this is all part of their self-soothing process. So, I think this is a good investment and, rather than making you over attentive, I think it gives you the confidence to pause and give your baby an opportunity to settle.

" *Having a camera monitor has made me a much less jumpy mummy. With my first baby I think I used to disturb her by going to check on her unnecessarily each time she stirred or grumbled. The video gives me the confidence to wait and observe to see if my intervention is actually necessary.* "

Liz, mother of Harriet, aged 5 months

23. Twins, triplets and more

As a mother of triplets, I would say the key thing that worked for me was routine, routine, routine!

I belong to a very active and supportive group of triplet and quad mums, and depending on the birth weight of our babies, the majority of us have followed a 3–4-hourly feeding schedule, whether breast or bottle feeding. Babies can be fed in tandem or one after the other. Obviously if you have help it is much easier, but not all of us have that luxury so it can be quite a juggling act.

This system of scheduled feeding may not be right for you if you have babies of very different weights or with medical issues, in which case you will need to be guided by your paediatrician. It is helpful to keep a daily feed and sleep diary for each baby.

Try to create a consistent pattern of feeding and sleeping, and once they have reached a healthy weight – if your health visitor or paediatrician is in agreement – you can allow them to sleep for longer periods at night. If one wakes to feed, I would suggest you feed them all to keep them in a consistent pattern.

Establish a set bedtime for your babies and don't worry too much about them waking each other. Multiples generally don't seem to be bothered by their siblings' cries. Mine could certainly sleep through each other's cries, which always amazed me!

Parents of multiples often don't have the time or capability to rock or feed their babies to sleep, so their babies may learn to self-settle at an earlier age. Once babies self-settle they are more likely to drop their night feeds of their own accord as they learn to soothe themselves back to sleep between sleep cycles and only wake if they are genuinely hungry.

You can choose to sleep your multiples in the same cot (co-bedding) or allow them to sleep in separate cots in the same room. Research has shown that sleeping similarly sized multiples in the same cot can help them to synchronise their sleep cycles. If you decide to co-bed, it is essential that you follow the safe co-bedding guidelines available through Twins Trust (www.twinstrust.org).

The early weeks will be very tiring so try to sleep when your babies sleep – even if you only have time for a 'power nap' in the day you will feel better for it. If your babies' cots don't fit in your room, set up a bed in their room and, if you have a partner, take turns doing the night feeds when possible.

Young babies can often get very fractious in the early evening, needing extra cuddles and soothing. If possible, try to get some help at this time; however, if you are alone, simple bouncy chairs are helpful as you can rock them with your feet while simultaneously soothing another baby. I personally wouldn't recommend the vibrating chairs as these can create an unhelpful sleep trigger/association.

Try to get out at least once a day, as light and fresh air help to develop your babies' biological day/night cycles. I don't think I left the house for the first month, but after that my afternoon stroll with my babies was my absolute sanity saver!

Caring for multiples is exhausting, so do accept offers of help and don't try to go it alone. Local colleges may offer childcare students on placement. I couldn't have managed without student help. There is also a charity called Homestart that can offer help and support in some parts of the country (www.home-start.org.uk).

My triplets were born at 35 weeks, we came out of hospital 12 days later and, by this time, I was feeding every 3 hours. They were very sleepy, so it wasn't difficult to establish this. I breastfed two of them fully and one had breast milk supplemented with formula due to weight loss. I breastfed to a schedule as I felt that this was the only way I could manage to feed them all. They became very proficient feeders, so naturally moved on to feeding approximately every 4 hours and it's ingrained in my mind that I fed them at 10, 2 and 6, both a.m. and p.m. I wasn't encouraged to breastfeed by the health professionals in hospital, I was even told that it wasn't possible to breastfeed triplets – however, I had done my research and I knew it was possible. I had one very supportive nurse in the special care unit who said if I was going to do this I needed to teach my babies to feed to a schedule and take their feed quickly! She was right. For us, this worked and it was a very positive experience. The babies' rhythms were governed by their feeding schedule and I could almost set my clock to the 2 a.m. feed. At night my husband would get the babies up, change nappies if necessary, and I would stay in bed and feed – the first two in tandem and then the third. We got so proficient at doing the night feed that we could have them all fed and back to sleep within the hour! This type of spaced feeding is certainly not right for all babies, but this is what worked in our situation.

24. Early rising

I feel the need to dedicate a section to early rising, as it is a common problem that can be exhausting for parents and one that can be difficult to resolve.

Once your baby has reached 6 months of age, I would suggest that you treat any time before 6 a.m. as night-time, depending on what time your baby goes to sleep at the start of the night. However, if your baby is regularly waking at 5 a.m. and not settling back to sleep you need to try to establish the reason for this.

There are four common reasons for early rising. These are:

1. Baby is being rewarded for early waking and will therefore persist in waking as they enjoy the contact – Rewards can come in various shapes, which are listed below, however, please remember that if what you are doing is working for you there is no need to make changes.

★ **Feeding at the early wake-up time, which can become a learnt hunger and perpetuate the early waking.**

SOLUTION – Avoid feeding at this time and instead use one of the settling techniques described in sections 22 and 27.

★ **Giving them your full attention at that time, so as not to disturb the rest of the family.**

SOLUTION – As you have read earlier, minimal attention is more effective at night-time. You need to leave your baby to entertain themself and, if you are consistent, they will learn that their waking will not be rewarded. Once you have reached an acceptable wake-up time, go to them and, using your happy daytime voice, open the curtains, make a fuss of them and start the day.

★ **Taking them into bed with you, so as not to disturb the rest of the family. This is a fabulous reward for early rising so your baby will definitely continue to do so!**

SOLUTION – You need to stop taking your baby into your bed and help them to resettle by using the techniques described above. Be prepared – your baby may protest, as you have previously showed them that the more they protest, the more likely you are to reward them. If you are consistent they will learn that their early waking will not be rewarded and they will gradually start to sleep later. If necessary, you may need to use a settling technique from sections 22 and 27, or with an older baby you may leave them to protest, maybe with a couple of soft toys to entertain them. This will call for a little tough love and some disturbed mornings for all the family, but it will pay dividends in the long term.

2. Timing of daytime naps – If the first nap of the day is too early and too long, this will be compensating for the early rising. Ideally, if your baby is over 6 months old the first nap of the day will be around 9 a.m. and should be for around 45–60 minutes with a longer nap at lunchtime. If your baby is napping too early, rather than suddenly moving their nap forwards and risking them becoming overtired, move the morning nap forwards by 15 minutes every two days until you reach the desired time.

3. Early sleep phase – If your baby is going to sleep very early in the evening, they are likely to wake early in the morning. For example, if they go to sleep at 6 p.m. and wake at 5 a.m., they have achieved a solid 11 hours of sleep and are therefore unlikely to resettle easily. To help your baby to readjust their body clock you need to help them to shift this whole period of night-time sleep forwards. You are more likely to succeed if you do this gradually to allow their body clock to accommodate the change. A more desirable sleep phase would be 7 p.m. to

6 a.m., therefore move bedtime forwards by 15 minutes every couple of nights until you reach the desired time, moving meal times and daytime naps accordingly. It may take 2–4 weeks for their body clock to adjust.

4. Light – Ensure there is no daylight filtering around the side of the curtains as light suppresses the sleep hormone, melatonin, and will therefore contribute to early waking. It is worth investing in blackout blinds. Portable ones are also available and worth considering when going on holiday.

25. Times of change

There are many developmental changes and physical factors that can affect your baby's sleep. These are often referred to as 'sleep regressions', but actually they are a time of developmental progress for your child. You may have got into a lovely predictable routine and then it all changes. During these periods of intense development, you may need to spend more time settling your baby to help them to feel secure as they go through these developmental stages. For example:

★ **Growth spurts –** Your baby's sleeping and waking patterns are influenced by hunger as well as their circadian rhythm, so while they are going through a growth spurt they may wake more regularly to feed. Growth spurts can happen any time during the first year but common times are between 1–3 weeks, 6–8 weeks, 3 months, 6 months and 9 months.

★ **Circadian rhythm changes** – The circadian rhythm is the 24-hour sequence of biological cycles that influences patterns of sleeping, waking, rest, hunger, activity, body temperature and hormones. Various factors can affect this, such as the length of sleep cycles extending as your baby matures; your baby being able to sleep for longer periods without feeding; and the development of non-REM sleep.

★ **Teething** – This can be disruptive to sleep and some babies experience more discomfort than others. There are various things you can do to alleviate the pain and, along with traditional medication, there are homeopathic remedies available. To prevent your baby from becoming dependent on your prolonged presence at night, try to deal with them in a quiet and straightforward way, avoiding bringing them into bed with you, and aim to get your normal routine back on track as soon as possible. If this does cause sleep problems, you may have to follow a gradual retreat process when they are well again. See sections 22 and 27.

★ **Separation anxiety** – This can start between the ages of 6 and 12 months. However, if you stay with your baby while they fall asleep, they will become dependent on your presence, so a better solution is to return regularly to comfort and reassure them until they fall asleep. See Part Five: Sleep Solutions – 6 Months Plus.

★ **4-month sleep regression** – As your baby's brain matures, their sleep pattern will change. Because of this, at around 3–4 months many babies become more wakeful at night. This is commonly termed 'the 4-month sleep regression' but it is actually a developmental progression. This coincides with a time when babies often get distracted when feeding as they are more interested in the world around them. This can cause them to be hungrier at night. By following the tips and advice in this book you should hopefully avoid this sleep regression.

★ **Ability to stay awake at will** – Avoid putting stimulating toys in your baby's cot as this will perpetuate this problem.

★ **Gross motor skills development** – Ability to sit up/stand up/crawl. At around 8–12 months your baby's sleep may be disrupted when they start to move around their cot, roll over, sit up and, in particular, when they learn to stand up against the side of their cot. This is especially problematic when they can stand up but cannot lower themself back down again. Try to help them to develop this skill by playing some daytime games where they lift and lower themself. If you have to lay them down at night, keep interaction to a minimum to avoid this becoming a game.

★ **Change in circumstances** – External factors can also affect sleep, like a new sibling, moving house, going on holiday, particularly to a different time zone, starting nursery or going to a childminder. You may need to give your baby extra comfort at these times and, once they are settled, gradually withdraw your presence. See Part Five: Sleep Solutions – 6 Months Plus.

★ **Clock change** – This is a time that many parents dread, particularly in the autumn when the clocks go back, which can cause an early riser to wake even earlier! You can either choose to 'go with the flow' and allow your baby or child's body clock to adapt naturally, or you can tweak your baby's schedule ahead of time. You do this by pushing bedtime forwards or backwards by 15 minutes every few days until bedtime has moved by one hour, and hopefully the wake-up time will adapt accordingly. You will also need to adjust naps, meal and milk times during the day.

★ **Illness** – If your baby is sleeping in their own bedroom and you need to monitor them due to illness, it is better to move a mattress onto the floor of their room, rather than bring them into your room to sleep. This will help avoid confusion and, once they are better, it will be easier to get back on track with their normal routine.

During times of change it can be really helpful to keep a sleep diary as this will help you to understand your baby's rhythms and you can adjust their routine accordingly. When you are writing a sleep diary, it is particularly useful to note how long it takes your baby to get to sleep. It should take no longer than 10–20 minutes. If it takes longer they may be under-tired or overtired and the easiest way to understand this is to look back over your diary to see what timings seem to be working best for your baby. There is a sleep diary template on pages 150–51 that you can use to copy and fill in.

Part Four:
SLEEP SUMMARY – NEWBORN TO 6 MONTHS

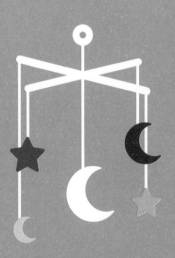

Now that you have read about how your baby sleeps and how to establish positive sleep habits, I thought it would be useful to recap on key points at different stages.

0-6 weeks

★ Anything goes! This is your time for bonding with your baby, getting to know each other and establishing feeding. If you are breastfeeding you will need to feed regularly to establish your milk supply.

★ Your newborn baby will not be able to self-settle so will need to be soothed. Some babies need a lot more pacifying than others in these early days.

★ Don't even think about 'sleep training'. In the early weeks, the key to a settled baby is a good feeding rhythm, so focus on 'making every feed count'. If your baby is hungry they will be unsettled.

★ Even though it's lovely to cuddle a sleeping baby, occasionally try to put your baby down in their Moses basket or cot, drowsy but awake enough to be aware of their surroundings.

★ Try not to over-stimulate your newborn baby. In the first month, the longest time your baby should be awake between naps is 45–60 minutes. Over-stimulation in the early weeks is common, causing your baby to be fractious, and can sometimes be misinterpreted as colic. Lots of visitors, being handed from person to person, much interaction and being rocked and jiggled can cause over-stimulation of your baby's sensory nervous system. You may need to consider sending your visitors home and taking your baby to a darkened room to gently soothe and calm them.

★ Help your baby to distinguish between night and day – see section 14.

6–12 weeks

★ Work on the timings of your feeds, whether breast- or bottle-feeds. Try to establish an organised but flexible feeding and sleeping routine based around your baby's own rhythms. If you are breastfeeding, encourage your baby to 'actively' feed. This should enable them to be settled and content for longer between feeds.

★ Adjust your routine, so you don't feed your baby just before they are due a nap or you will create a sleep association and your baby will only know how to go to sleep while feeding. This may result in total dependence and regular night waking in the future.

★ Feeding your baby after a nap will also ensure that they have the energy to take a bigger feed.

★ Continue to help your baby to distinguish between night and day.

★ Try to implement the 'pause'. Observe and listen to your baby.

★ Establish a bath and bedtime routine.

★ Help your baby to self-settle for naps and at night-time try to put them to bed drowsy but awake enough to be aware of their surroundings. Try to avoid feeding them to sleep.

★ Use the same sleep cue words each time you put your baby down for a sleep.

3–6 months

★ Some babies may sleep through the night at 3 months and some may still be waking for one or two feeds at night at 6 months. All babies are unique and have different needs. Don't compare your baby with your friend's baby.

★ If you haven't already implemented a regular bath routine, now is the time to do so.

★ If your feeds are close together, increase the intervals between feeds gradually. If your baby is taking a bigger feed they will be more satisfied and will sleep for longer periods.

★ Establish a regular daytime pattern of feeding and napping, and avoid feeding your baby just before a sleep.

★ Encourage your baby to self-settle, night and day.

★ Consider giving the final feed of the day, just before a bath, to disassociate feeding and sleeping, or offer a split feed either side of the bath.

★ Try to avoid feeding to sleep – this is key!

★ At 6 months, if your baby is healthy and eating well during the day, but still waking for regular night feeds, you can start to gradually wean them off.

Part Five:
SLEEP SOLUTIONS - 6 MONTHS PLUS

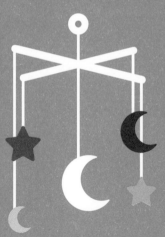

26. Have you missed the early boat?

I encourage all parents to establish positive sleep habits early on, however it's never too late to help your baby to sleep better – so if you have just picked up this book and your baby is over 6 months old, this part is for you.

If you haven't helped your baby to settle independently from a young age you need to prepare yourself for a bit of a bumpy ride. Well-established sleep habits will take time to change, so consistency is vital.

The crying debate

A cause of great confusion and angst among parents is whether it is detrimental to their baby's emotional well-being to allow them to cry. I feel this is an issue that is often taken out of context and misrepresented in many debates, particularly on the Internet.

My view on crying in general is that allowing your baby to cry a little is a way of respecting their voice and allowing them to communicate with you. If you immediately quell every cry, you are missing the opportunity to listen to their voice, and yourself time to try to interpret and respond to their needs.

There are some very strong opinions regarding crying, some that may scare parents into thinking they should **never** allow their baby to cry. However, sometimes your baby needs to have a grizzle and a groan to get themselves off to sleep or in between sleep cycles during the night. I advocate simply not responding too quickly when your baby stirs, allow a little time unless you think that there is something wrong or your baby's cry tells you there is.

I absolutely think that you should respond to your baby and that if they are distressed, they are trying to tell you that they have needs that must be met. Pausing and listening does not mean that you are being unresponsive – quite the opposite. Taking time to understand your baby and responding with the appropriate action – whether it's food, touch or warmth – is positive parenting. Sometimes you may find that having cuddled, rocked and jiggled your baby and found that nothing is calming them, putting them down in their crib or on their play mat is the answer. Sometimes babies just need a bit of space and calm as they are over-stimulated.

There are strongly conflicting opinions about sleep-training methods that involve leaving your baby to cry and none of these methods should be considered for a baby under 6 months old. There is the school of thought that says that conditioning your baby not to cry by not meeting their needs can result in psychological damage. However, we have other sleep doctors stating that long-term sleep deprivation is physically and psychologically damaging, to both the child and their carers, and that using a sleep-training technique is healthier than continuing this damaging cycle.

I regularly work with families whose babies are sleep deprived and waking between every sleep cycle during the night as they cannot get themselves back to sleep without help. This also causes the baby to become fretful during the day and, for a sleep-deprived parent, this is not a healthy situation to be in. The parent may then not be able to make positive parental decisions and may make poor judgements due to their exhaustion. This can have a negative effect on all members of the family. It's a vicious circle, as the more tired a baby is the more difficult they will find it to get to sleep. Therefore, helping your baby to sleep is essential in this situation but should be carried out in a way that meets your baby's needs and offers reassurance.

Leaving your baby to cry for hours on end, day after day or night after night, is no doubt damaging, but this should not be confused with using a technique where your baby is comforted with your presence or offered frequent reassurance. Helping to improve your baby's sleep using gentle methods can provide a long-term solution and should not be confused with neglecting your baby's needs. Long-term sleep deprivation can have a significant effect on a child's behaviour and their ability to learn, so it's important to address this.

Checklist

Before embarking on any settling techniques, it is crucial that you have all the building blocks in place, so go through the following checklist first. You may even find that focusing on some of the below points resolves your baby's sleep issues without the need for further intervention.

Is your baby getting plenty of exposure to daylight and fresh air?
Getting your baby out into the daylight as early as possible in the mornings and reducing exposure to light in the evenings will help regulate melatonin production and reinforce the difference between night and day.

Is your baby getting enough age-appropriate exercise?
Give opportunities for babies to roll, sit, crawl, bounce and walk with support.

Is your baby taking regular daytime naps?
Sleep encourages sleep. In order for your baby to sleep well at night they need to be well rested. If a baby is

overtired their body will produce the hormone cortisol to help them cope with the fatigue. This gives a 'second wind' effect, makes it harder for your baby to go to sleep, and may result in regular night waking and early rising. Work on encouraging good daytime naps. If your baby is taking lots of short naps, gradually space the time between them and try to get your baby to have at least one nap a day in their cot,

Is your daytime routine consistent?
Making the timings of your baby's meals, naps, wake-up time and bedtime consistent will help to regulate their circadian rhythm (body clock) and should make settling easier.

Is your baby watching TV before bedtime?
Avoid exposure to screens and TV particularly in the 2 hours before bedtime as the blue light emitted inhibits the production of melatonin.

Do you have a regular, predictable bath routine?
See section 20. This will help your baby to produce the hormone melatonin, which helps regulate sleep/wake cycles. It also provides sleep cues, which help the baby to expect sleep.

Have you tried using white or pink noise at nap and sleep times?

This background noise can calm babies, helping them to fall asleep quicker and stay asleep by masking distractive noises such as traffic, household sounds or sibling and parental noise. Be sure to keep it on all night though!

Is your baby eating well during the day?

You can't expect your baby to sleep well if they are hungry! Make sure they are taking regular milk feeds during the day with good intervals in between to encourage them to take a bigger and more satisfying feed. If they are over 6 months encourage a nutritious, well-balanced diet so they are not hungry during the night. Certain foods are reported to be sleep inducing, particularly cherries, bananas, warm milk, cottage cheese, yogurt, eggs, chicken, turkey, sweet potatoes, oats and cereals.

Is your baby in good health?

If you have any doubts, seek advice from your GP, health visitor or paediatrician.

Does your baby have a 'sleep association'? What is it?

If your baby is feeding to sleep it would be beneficial to reorganise your routine so that a feed doesn't come just before sleep. Your baby may find it difficult to fall asleep at first as they don't know how to without feeding. You may need to do a lot of soothing, and to begin with you can even go for long walks or take them for a drive to help them to nap. Initially it doesn't matter what you do or how you do it, just focus on not feeding to sleep. The next step will be to move on to one of the settling methods explained below.

27. Techniques to help your baby learn to settle independently

It is unfair to attempt any of these methods before the above building blocks are in place. Go through the checklist above before you commence, then:

★ Choose one of the sleep-solution methods below and start at night-time as your baby's melatonin levels will be higher in the evening, so this should help them to settle easier.

★ Choose the solution that feels most comfortable for you and stay with it; don't change tack after a few days as you will confuse your baby.

★ Ensure that both you and your partner are in agreement. Two teachers are better than one.

★ The gentler techniques tend to take longer and need lots of patience, but involve less crying. Choose a time to start when you can stick to a consistent routine, i.e. not just before you are going on holiday.

★ Choose a time when your baby is well and you are well.

★ Ensure your baby has a full tummy, ideally having their last feed before your short and soothing bath routine, or a split feed either side of their bath

★ Be consistent and do not make a half-hearted attempt. It's unfair on you and your baby and may make the situation worse.

Gradual retreat

This is my favoured method. It is a gentle technique whereby you gradually move on to the next degree of separation. Your starting point will be governed by what your baby has become dependent on.

★ If your baby has always fed to sleep, keep an eye out for when they stop actively feeding and move them away from their milk source when they have. If you are breastfeeding, try to unlatch them when they have stopped vigorously sucking. The easiest way to do this is to gently insert your finger into the corner of their mouth to break the suction and remove your nipple from their mouth. Your baby will probably root and cry as they have previously been allowed to stay sucking as an aid to get to sleep. Try to cuddle and calm your baby. If you need to allow them to feed again, do exactly the same thing, when they have finished sucking vigorously, unlatch from the breast or remove bottle, calm and cuddle them. Repeat, as necessary. We want them to be sleepy but not asleep.

★ When they have learnt to fall asleep without sucking, you can move on to the next step of settling them in their cot when they are drowsy. Your baby may find it easier to get to sleep if your partner or someone who is not breastfeeding settles them to avoid associating food with sleep.

★ If you have always rocked your baby to sleep in your arms now is the time to move to the next degree of separation, which is laying them in their cot and helping them to settle with your presence.

★ After a cuddle, settle your baby into their cot saying, 'It's sleep time now' and your reassuring sleep cue words.

★ Stay with your baby, soothe them, gently pat, shush and encourage them to sleep. Sometimes shushing loudly can distract your baby from crying.

★ Avoid engaging with them. Be boring! However long your baby tries to fight sleep, the most important thing is that you see this through until sleep is achieved. Stay with them. It may take some time at first as they will expect to be picked up, especially if they've learnt to fall asleep in your arms, so they need to understand what you are expecting of them.

★ Try not to pick your baby up and cuddle them, try to give them comfort and reassurance while in their cot. You may need to lean over and almost cuddle them in their cot. However, if they are inconsolable and you feel it is necessary, give them a cuddle until they calm down and then start the process again making sure they go back in their cot awake.

★ Your aim is to help them to go to sleep without your intervention. With a gradual retreat process you will move on to the next degree of separation once they have gone to sleep two or three times in this way and when the time taken to achieve sleep has shortened.

★ Do not leave the room until you are sure they are soundly asleep. Wait at least 10 minutes as leaving too early when they may only be partially asleep may disturb them and you may have to start all over again!

★ The next step would be to give less help and intervention, therefore you may give just an occasional pat, shush or put a reassuring firm hand on their back, again staying with them until they fall asleep.

★ After a couple of successes with this, you may just sit on the floor next to their cot, and once you think they are ready and comfortable falling asleep independently, move completely away once you have settled them.

★ With this method you need to observe, listen and judge when it is time to move on to the next degree of separation, you may even find that your presence is over-stimulating and interferes with your baby going to sleep, in which case, it's time to step back.

★ Another starting point that some parents feel comfortable with is laying, with eyes closed, on a camp bed next to their baby's cot. Even though their baby may be crying, they are by their side.

★ Whichever starting point you choose, you must keep your goal in mind, which is to give less and less intervention over a period of time and distance yourself until your baby is comfortable to settle alone.

★ This is a trust technique and will take time and patience. You are giving the message that you are there for them and will respond when they cry, but you do expect them to go to sleep in their cot. By offering them comfort and reassurance, you are modelling the behaviour that a baby or child should follow in terms of how to soothe themself.

★ This method will work but you must see it through and be 100 per cent consistent.

★ Each time your baby goes to sleep in this way, it will be easier for them the next time.

★ Don't try any method two or three times and then give up just as you were about to turn the corner. KEEP GOING!

Pick up and put down

If you do not feel ready for gradual retreat, then this could be the method for you. After following your usual routine, lay your baby in their cot, drowsy but awake, saying your soothing sleep cue words. If they cry and cannot be calmed, pick them up and comfort them until they are calm and drowsy but not asleep. Put them back in their cot and repeat this cycle as many times as necessary until they are asleep. This technique will build trust and gives your baby the reassurance that you are there for them. It requires time and patience, but for some older babies the picking up and putting down may be over-stimulating.

Once your baby has learnt to go to sleep in this way, continue with gradual retreat, as above.

Check and console

Although I favour gradual retreat, check and console can work more quickly if you are consistent, but this method may involve more crying. For parents of multiples sometimes this is the only practical solution if their babies or toddlers are sharing a room. Only use it with a baby over 6 months old, who is from a safe, secure and loving background. It is not suitable for babies with a highly sensitive temperament.

Timed method

When following this technique, it is important to show your baby that you are being responsive to their needs by returning and providing love, reassurance, and giving them clear and gentle explanations of what you expect of them. I will give you an example of timings, but you can of course adapt this to suit you and your baby.

Night one:

★   **After your usual calming bedtime routine, give your baby a cuddle, settle them into their cot saying** 'it's sleep time now' and use your reassuring sleep cue words.

★ As you leave the room, you could say something like, 'I'm just going to the toilet and I'll be right back.' They may cry.

★ Wait for 1 minute. Then go back in for up to 2 minutes, and comfort and reassure by laying your hand on them saying, 'Shush, shush, there, there, it's sleep time now.' You can give them a kiss if you want, there are no hard and fast rules. Do what you feel comfortable with.

★ Leave the room for 2 minutes, again saying that you'll be back soon, and once again return to give comfort and reassurance for up to 1-2 minutes.

★ Continue this process, increasing the time of absence in 1-minute increments, building up to 5 minutes spent out of the room on the first night. Repeat this process until they are asleep, however long it takes!

★ If your older baby stands against the side of their cot, gently lay them down saying it's sleep time and avoid any further engagement.

Night two:

★ Start with 2 minutes out of the room and up to 2 minutes in, building up to 6 minutes out of the room.

Night three:

★ **Start with 3 minutes out of the room and up to 1 minute in, building up to 8 minutes out of the room.**

Night four (if necessary!)

★ **Start with 4 minutes out of the room and up to 1 minute in, building up to 10 minutes out of the room.**

★ **Repeat night four timings for subsequent nights, if necessary.**

Each time you return to the room the intention is to give reassurance rather than get your baby to sleep. The most important thing is to listen to their cries. If they are just grizzling or the volume of their cry is reducing, you do not need to go back to them, or you may disturb their self-settling process. Only go back and reassure if you think their crying is escalating into distress.

If you prefer not to watch the clock, you can follow the same process but return to reassure your baby at more randomly spaced intervals depending on the sound of their cries, especially if you find that your reassurances are antagonising them more.

If your baby becomes overly distressed, you may need to pick them up and calm them, but try not to allow them to fall asleep in your arms. When they are calm, put them back in the cot and start again.

This is a learning process, your baby may cry and shout with anger and frustration as they are not sure what is expected of them – they've never done it before! You are teaching them that you expect them to go to sleep in their cot while giving them regular reassurances so they do not feel abandoned. They will get the message if you are consistent. Try to interpret their cries, and assess when you need to go in and reassure. Remember that even babies who self-settle and sleep well often take 20 minutes to get to sleep, so make a cup of tea and prepare yourself – it may take some time.

Key points to remember:

★ Give yourself small, realistic goals.

★ Whichever method you choose, it is essential that you see it through until sleep is achieved. These methods do work if you are 100 per cent consistent. Do not give up after two or three tries. Your baby will be confused.

★ Prepare yourself – this can be exceptionally hard. No one likes to hear their baby cry, but you will be giving regular reassurances. Remind yourself why you are helping your baby to sleep; sleep deprivation can be damaging to the whole family.

★ With any change in routine, things can get worse before they get better.

★ Quite often, following a successful period, you may have a test night or two of regression. Be persistent and consistent and you should get back on track.

★ You need to send a clear message to your baby or toddler about what is expected, so whatever is happening at one sleep situation needs to happen for all sleep situations; night-time, nap times and if your baby or toddler wakes during the night.

★ Keep a sleep diary detailing what you do and how long it takes your baby to get to sleep. You should start to see improvements after 3-4 days. However, the older your baby is, the longer it may take, so do not give up, that would be unfair on your baby and make it doubly hard if you reattempt at another time.

★ Real change for regular improved nights and naps may take one week or may take three or four, depending on the method you choose and how quickly you progress with it. Putting the effort in now will pay dividends in the future.

★ Always put your baby down for sleeps before they get overtired, they will find it easier to settle. Look for sleep signs and keep a sleep diary to help you understand your baby's rhythms.

★ If your baby becomes unwell at all during this period, give them the comfort they need and then go back to it when they are well again.

* A baby's needs and sleep routine will change over time, so look for the signs of this and adapt your routine as necessary.
* If you have a bad day, put it behind you and move on. We all have bad days.
* Be positive! Don't dread putting your baby down for their sleep. They will sense your anxiety. Put them down to sleep in a positive way and fully expect them to sleep. When they learn to self-settle they will love going to sleep!

> Consistency is key!

" At 7 months old, our son was waking multiple times overnight and needed to be breastfed back to sleep. Consequently he was not interested in food during the day. We decided to use the gradual retreat technique and found that Jake responded well to me soothing him to sleep instead of my wife as he didn't associate me with food. He now sleeps through the night and is so much happier for it. "

Alex, father of Jake, 8 months

28. Baby sleep: solutions to common problems

My baby will only fall asleep on the breast or while bottle feeding...

Your baby has developed an association with feeding and sleeping. This is their cue for sleep so you need to introduce alternative sleep cues to help them learn to self-settle without this dependence. In the first 6–8 weeks, feeding them to sleep is positive as you are encouraging your baby to take big full feeds, so it's inevitable that they may fall asleep on the breast or bottle. However, even at this age try to occasionally put your baby down to sleep, drowsy but awake.

If your baby is older, avoid feeding just before your baby is due a sleep. You need to completely disassociate feeding and sleeping. A good daytime sleep/awake pattern to follow is: sleep, feed, play, repeat. Furthermore, this will encourage your baby to take a good, full feed as they won't be falling asleep while feeding. Refer to section 20 – Routine/feeding and napping.

If you are breastfeeding, your baby is likely to be using the nipple as a pacifier. This is a habit that many mothers find the most difficult to break. The first step is to start to unlatch your baby from the breast when they have finished actively feeding. If they root for the nipple again, then try to cuddle and soothe them. If they continue to root and cry, let them suck again if necessary, but repeat the same process, taking them off the breast as soon as they have finished actively feeding. Continue this process every time you feed.

I would suggest using a gradual retreat process to introduce different cues to help your baby to settle without feeding. See section 27 – Techniques to help your baby learn to settle independently.

Our baby will only fall asleep in our bed...

Babies learn by association so, if they have always fallen asleep in this way this is all they know. The earlier you teach your baby to self-settle in their own cot or Moses basket, the easier it will be. They may not like it to begin with, so choose a settling technique (see sections 22 and 27) and prepare to see it through however long it takes. You will be amazed how quickly your baby will learn if you do the same thing every time. Time, repetition and consistency are key. Another tip for the winter is to put a warm hot water bottle in their sleeping space and remove it before you place them in, just to take the chill off and make it a cosier place to be. Never use boiling water and always check the temperature before placing your child in the bed, it should be warm to the touch but not hot.

"Charlotte had never slept well and at 5 months old I could only get her to sleep in our bed at night and in my arms during the day. I was exhausted. Every time I put Charlotte in her cot she screamed but, in picking her up the whole time, I was inadvertently rewarding her cries and I didn't know what else to do. Stephanie taught me to soothe Charlotte in her cot, and she did cry for 35 minutes on the first day, but I stayed with her until sleep was achieved. This was the secret, to see it through, as every day the time got shorter and shorter. Within a week Charlotte was sleeping in her cot during the day and the following week during the night. I was determined not to make the same mistakes with our second baby and I started to teach her to self-settle from week one! She is a great sleeper. I just put her down in her cot and she goes to sleep. No props, just a soft cloth comforter."

Angela, mother of Charlotte and Savanna, now aged 4 years and 1 year

My baby won't settle...
Choose a settling technique that you are comfortable with and suits your parenting style. If you are consistent and do the same thing every time, your baby will learn to settle. If you try a new technique for only three times and then give up, you are sure to fail. Your baby will become confused as they have not had sufficient opportunity to learn a new behaviour and you will reinforce the crying. Time, repetition and consistency are key, otherwise you may give up just as your baby was starting to get the message and succeed.

It took me 40 minutes to settle my baby in his cot for a nap and then he only slept for half an hour...
If you are just embarking on helping them to establish new sleeping habits you may be more successful at bedtime as their melatonin levels will be higher in the evenings, inducing drowsiness and readiness for sleep.

Once your baby has mastered the art of self-settling his naps will become longer and longer. Consistency will pay off. If it's been difficult one day, don't try again on the same day, give yourself and your baby a break and take them out for a long walk or a drive instead. Be positive – tomorrow is a new day.

My 6-month-old baby is waking every 2–3 hours in the night...

This behaviour is usually due to your baby not settling independently at the start of the night. Babies rouse between sleep cycles and if your baby has become dependent on going to sleep with an inappropriate sleep association or prop they will struggle to connect their sleep cycles independently during these partial wakings. The most common sleep associations are feeding or rocking to sleep. Whatever it is, your baby will be dependent on it throughout the night. See section 15 – Sleep associations, and help your baby learn to self-settle using one of the techniques in section 27. Also look at their nap schedule to ensure that they are getting the correct amount of sleep at appropriate times during the day.

My baby will only catnap...

If your baby is self-settling this should improve as they become more proficient at connecting their sleep cycles. From around 6 months you are aiming for two to three naps during the day with the longest one being at lunchtime, so if this continues to be short, take a look at your routine and timings. An ideal routine at this age would be a 45–60-minute nap in the morning, 1.5–2 hours around lunchtime and a short nap before teatime so your baby is not overtired at bath time.

If the situation doesn't improve, but if your baby sleeps well in the pushchair, you could try taking them for a long walk in the middle of the day with the aim of getting them to sleep for at least two sleep cycles (1.5 hours). Do this for four or five days. The aim of this will be to get their body used to sleeping for the longer period. Then return to midday cot naps and hopefully they will find it easier to connect their sleep cycles.

Another trick is to wait outside their room at around the time they usually wake. As soon as they stir, go in and do anything that will help them get back to sleep. Rub their tummy, shush, pat. This is a time to ignore the usual rules and help them to resettle. Repeat as necessary, to help them achieve a longer nap.

My 8-month-old baby is waking at 5 a.m. and then having a 2-hour early morning nap...

This long early morning nap is perpetuating the early rising. Gradually move the morning nap forwards in 15-minute increments until you reach 9 a.m. and gradually shorten the length of it to no longer than 1 hour. Aim for your baby's long nap to be at lunchtime.

My 4-month-old baby is feeding every 2 hours...

If there is no medical reason why your baby should feed so regularly, gradually increase the time between feeds. For the first couple of days feed every 2.25 hours, for the second couple of days feed every 2.5 hours and so on until you are feeding every 3–4 hours. You will need to keep your baby occupied and distracted to elongate the time between feeds. Over time they should start to take a bigger feed and this will satisfy them for longer periods between feeds. If you are breastfeeding ensure that you have a good, deep latch and that your baby is 'actively' feeding as babies can get very distracted at this age.

My daughter is 6.5 months old and I would really like to establish a regular routine for her. Can you help?
A typical routine at this age would be as follows, but remember all babies are unique so keep a sleep diary, and try to adopt a routine that suits your baby's rhythms and fits in with your lifestyle.

7 a.m.: Awake. Breast- or bottle-feed followed by breakfast.

9–9.30 a.m.: Nap – one sleep cycle – 45–60 minutes. Breast- or bottle-feed on waking, if needed.

11.30 a.m.–12 p.m.: Lunch.

12–12.30 p.m.: Long nap – ideally at least two sleep cycles – 1.5–2 hours.

2.30–3 p.m.: Breast- or bottle-feed.

4–4.30 p.m.: Short nap of 30–45 minutes (depending on earlier naps). Babies don't usually settle well in their cots for this late-afternoon nap, so maybe go for a walk. We don't want her to be too tired at bedtime or she will fall asleep during her pre-bath feed.

5 p.m.: Dinner.

6.15 p.m.: Breast- or bottle-feed.

6.30 p.m.: Bath, followed by a small top-up feed if necessary, but avoid feeding to sleep.

7 p.m.: Sleep.

I give my baby a dream feed at 10 p.m. but he still wakes 2 hours later...

I would suggest that you stop dream feeding and allow your baby to regulate his own body clock. During the first part of the night your baby is most likely to be in a deep sleep so it's best to avoid stimulating his digestive system at this time if he's not showing signs of hunger. You may find that he sleeps for a much longer stretch without the dream feed. See section 19 – Feeding at night.

My baby keeps losing her dummy in the night...

People often ask me my thoughts on dummies. If using a dummy works for you and your baby then it's fine, but if it's causing a problem and contributing to night-time waking, you either need to consider weaning your baby off it, or if they are old enough, encourage them to replace it themself. Putting extra dummies in the cot will make them easier to find. Alternatively, you can purchase soft cloth toys with Velcro to attach the dummies to, making them easier for small hands to find in the night. Ensure any toys that go in the cot are age appropriate, with a CE mark showing they have been tested to the necessary specifications for your baby's age.

My baby has started to stand up in her cot...

This can be a particular problem when your baby does not know how to lower themself. Practise during the daytime by playing pulling up and lowering back down games. It can be most frustrating when you lower your baby at night and she stands straight back up again, but be careful not to turn this into a game!

My baby is 8 months old and still waking for a night feed...

If your baby is in good health and eating well during the day, you can wean them off this feed. If they are breastfed, gradually reduce the number of minutes you offer each night. When they have got used to taking a very small amount, stop offering milk and use one of the settling techniques. See section 27 – Techniques to help your baby learn to settle independently

If your baby is bottle fed, reduce the volume of milk you give them gradually over a number of nights. Once your baby is used to taking a smaller amount, stop offering a bottle and use one of the settling techniques. At this age you can offer water instead of milk, however you may find that your baby still wakes to suck for comfort.

My 5-month-old son has been sleeping through until 4 a.m. for the past month and has recently started waking at 12.30 a.m. Should I feed him then?
Don't automatically assume that your son needs a feed at that time. Try to settle him back to sleep without feeding, if he is genuinely hungry he will not settle and will be sure to let you know. In which case, he may be going through a growth spurt.

My 9-month-old twins are rocked to sleep in their bouncy chairs and then we lift them into their cots, but they are repeatedly waking in the night and are difficult to resettle...
Your babies need to learn to settle to sleep in their cots. When they rouse between sleep cycles in the night, they are finding themselves in a different place to where they fell asleep and do not know how they got there, which

can be confusing and may make them feel insecure. In addition to this they do not know how to get themselves back to sleep without being rocked.

Part Six:
CASE
STUDIES

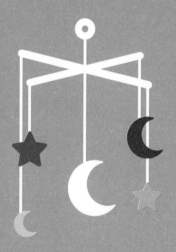

Willow – 16 weeks old

Situation – Willow's parents contacted me as Willow was waking repeatedly during the night, literally every hour. Both parents were exhausted and hadn't achieved more than 3 hours total sleep at night for the previous few weeks. Each time Willow woke at night she was fed or rocked back to sleep. During the evening she slept in Mum or Dad's arms until they went to bed and then she was put into her cot when she was soundly sleeping. During the day she was fed or rocked to sleep in her bouncy chair. The night before I met the family, Willow had woken eight times between midnight and 5 a.m. and had then slept in the parents' bed through their desperation to get a little more sleep!

Comments – Willow had never fallen asleep independently, which resulted in her waking every time she roused during the night and needing to be fed or rocked back to sleep again. She also had no night-time routine to help her to differentiate night and day.

Solution – Firstly, I reassured Willow's parents that this was a normal baby sleep pattern. As Willow was so young, my advice to her parents was to establish some positive habits to help the situation and to minimise future sleep problems, but she was too young for 'sleep training'. I advised them to establish a short, predictable bath routine, commencing around 6.30 p.m., offering

Willow a split feed, half before her bath and a top-up after, and then helping her to self-settle in her cot by using a gradual retreat process, or pick-up, put-down process as necessary.

During the day, the parents were asked to help Willow to settle in any way that didn't involve the feeding-to-sleep association. Initially, this might be going for a walk or rocking, and once night times had improved they could work on settling her into her cot in the daytime.

Outcome – As Willow had never gone to sleep in her cot before, she needed a lot of soothing and comfort to begin with. On the first night she, of course, cried as she didn't know what was expected of her, but she was picked up and cuddled until she was calm, and then put down and shushed and comforted in her cot. Mum said that at times she was almost cuddling Willow in her cot while stroking her head gently and saying reassuring gentle words. Mum used long and short shushing sounds, and when Willow was really worked up she gently rolled her on her side and patted her back until the crying had subsided. This proved effective for Willow. In these early days you do whatever works to soothe to sleep and pick up only when necessary.

On the first night Willow took 49 minutes to get to sleep, however Mum stayed by her side for the whole time and consoled and reassured her. On this very first night she only woke once at 2.15 a.m. and had a breastfeed, settled back to sleep and then woke again at 3.20 a.m., when Mum was able to soothe her back to sleep without lifting her. She woke for the day at 6.30 a.m. An amazing first night!

On night two, Willow took 31 minutes to get to sleep and on night three, 24 minutes. As time went on Willow took less and less time to get to sleep, and Mum and Dad worked on gradually retreating to the next degree of separation by using less interaction and soothing.

From the very start of the new routine Willow only woke once or twice during the night. She was at the perfect age to introduce new sleep cues and enjoyed her new bath time routine. She did start waking early in the morning, but instead of bringing her into their bed, which would reinforce the waking, her parents soothed her and gave her comfort in her cot.

Willow's parents also 'paused' in the night when she stirred as they understood that, in order for her to learn to connect her sleep cycles, they had to give her the opportunity to do so. They had previously been picking her up every time she made a noise, possibly waking her unnecessarily.

Once the night-time sleeping had improved they focused their attention on getting a daytime feeding and napping routine in place, and worked on Willow having at least one nap a day in her cot.

Mum's comments:

'One of the most valuable things you have taught me is simply to "allow Willow her voice". Before you said that to me, I was always desperate to find the quickest way to stop her from crying. Now I understand that sometimes she just needs a little cry and I've learnt to differentiate her cries much better.

'You have literally transformed our lives so we can all sleep again! I can now put Willow down to sleep in the evening, stand back (out of her eyeline), watch her grizzle and groan for 10 minutes and then fall asleep. I rather like this bit of the day, watching my baby fall asleep!'

Tamara – 12 months old

Situation – Early rising. Tamara had learnt to self-settle and generally went to bed at about 7 p.m., but woke at 5 a.m., just a little too early to start the day. Mum and Dad had tried feeding her and putting her back to bed, but she wouldn't settle so they started the day. However, this meant that Tamara was tired again by 7 a.m. and would go back down for a 1.5–2-hour nap. She would then have another shorter nap around lunchtime and would still be tired in the evening. Her parents had also tried putting her to bed later in the hope that she would wake later, but this was unsuccessful.

Comments – Typical sleep requirements at this age are approximately 11 hours at night (but 12, if you are lucky) and 2–2.5 hours during the day. The longer nap should be around lunchtime, but should not go past 3–3.30 p.m. Early rising is very common and often the most difficult situation to deal with as your baby has had a good chunk of sleep and is feeling revitalised even if you are not! Early rising is usually perpetuated by the following: rewarding the waking, learnt hunger or wrongly scheduled naps. In Tamara's case all three of these were happening. Tamara was allowed to start the day at 5 a.m. and enjoyed the attention given to her at this time. She also had a feed then, so had learnt to be hungry at that time and she was napping too early, thereby the first nap of the day was really a part of the night-time sleep that had become disjointed from the rest of the night. She was also overtired by the time she went to bed in the evening, which causes the body to produce the hormone cortisol, which can perpetuate early rising.

Solution – The parents were advised firstly to ensure a regular predictable night-time bed/bath routine. The morning nap needed to be shifted forwards and shortened as this was allowing Tamara to compensate for the lack of night-time sleep. If it was shifted forward too quickly Tamara would get overtired so her parents were advised to move this nap forward slowly in 15-minute increments until they reached 9 a.m. and to gradually shorten this nap to a maximum of 1 hour. The morning feed was also moved forward in 15-minute increments until Tamara's first feed of the day was at 6.30 a.m. When Tamara woke early her parents were advised to leave her to play/cry in her cot until the agreed time each day.

Outcome – On day one, Tamara woke at 5 a.m. as usual. She was left for 15 minutes, in which time she did cry but was not overly distressed. The following day her parents did not go to her until 5.15 a.m. once again, and the subsequent two days she was left until 5.30 a.m. and so on. Every two days the time before her parents entered her room extended by 15 minutes. During this time her morning nap was also shifted forward slowly and although she was tired she was not left to get overtired. She was not happy about being left to her own devices in the mornings, but she had some soft toys in her cot and soon learnt that her waking wouldn't be rewarded.

Her wake-up time gradually moved forwards, but it took about 4 weeks before her wake-up time adjusted to 6–6.30 a.m. With some babies it may take a week and with others it may take a month, but if you are consistent the situation will improve.

Another point to consider if you have an early riser is that your baby's bedtime may be too late! I know this sounds crazy, but it's true. If a baby goes to bed with high cortisol levels because they are overtired, they will find it more difficult to go to sleep, may be unsettled during the night and are more likely to wake early. Slowly bring their bedtime forwards.

Another common reason for early rising is that the parents bring the baby/child into their bed in order to get some more precious sleep themselves. When you are exhausted you will do anything for a little more sleep, but this reinforces the behaviour. Of course your baby will wake early for this special treat and the waking time will probably get earlier and earlier. You have to work through this so you all can benefit from a full night's sleep. Make a plan and be consistent!

Mum's comments:

'Stephanie explained to us from the start that early rising is one of the most common situations and one of the trickiest to resolve. However, I'm so pleased we worked through it, as starting the day at 5 a.m. was beginning to take its toll! Alongside that, I am going back to work shortly and Tamara's early rising and subsequent long morning nap just would not fit in with day care.'

Oliver – 11 months old

Situation – Repeated night waking, unsettled in the early evening and very little daytime sleep.

Oliver's parents had followed 'attachment parenting' with Oliver as he was very unsettled as a young baby. He co-slept at night and, during the day, they carried him in a sling, where he would have his daytime naps. This had worked quite well when he was younger but at 11 months old he was a big boy and was too heavy to carry in a sling for long periods. He therefore had daytime naps in his pushchair or in the car as he had never slept in a cot. At night his mum would breastfeed him to sleep and he would settle in the parental bed, but would wake up repeatedly until his parents came to bed and would wake regularly during the night to feed. He was often overtired during the day and his parents were exhausted too as a result of continually disturbed sleep.

As a sleep consultant, I always follow the parents' wishes and offer solutions that the parents feel comfortable with. In Oliver's case, the parents were clear from the start that they did not want to consider 'controlled crying' or similar and that they ideally wanted to continue to co-sleep.

Comments – When a baby rouses during the night in between sleep cycles, they need to find themselves in exactly the same situation as they fell asleep in. They will then feel safe and able to connect to their next sleep cycle.

In Oliver's case he was falling asleep while nursing, lying down with Mum and sometimes with Dad as well. When he was asleep they would creep downstairs, he would miss their presence when he roused and subsequently wake up again. During the night he needed Mum to nurse him back to sleep between sleep cycles as he had never learnt to connect his sleep cycles independently. The regular night feeds were sometimes causing him to open his bowels in the night and also affecting his daytime appetite. At his age, Oliver did not require night feeds for nourishment as he had a good diet during the day. Daytime sleep was a particular issue as Oliver needed to learn to sleep in a cot in order to achieve good physiologically restorative sleep in a safe environment.

Solution – We had no plans for a quick-fix solution with Oliver, just a gentle step-by-step approach. Our first aim was to disassociate feeding and sleeping so, during the first week the parents were asked to follow a regular bath routine with Oliver. Then Mum breastfed him in a chair, but didn't allow him to fall asleep while nursing. Then Mum or Dad would lay with Oliver in the parental bed, soothing him as necessary until he was asleep. If he woke before the parents came to bed, Mum or Dad would lay with him again and soothe or cuddle him without feeding. After the first week Mum and Dad were asked to give less and less intervention to help Oliver get to sleep, so instead of cuddling to sleep, they were to just lay by his side without giving eye contact or interacting with him, and then after a few days, lay with their backs to him and then gradually move to the edge of the bed, eventually just sitting on the side of the bed. I also asked for just one parent to be with him as they had both previously been present when he went to sleep.

Once Oliver had learnt to go to sleep without nursing we needed to teach him to sleep in his cot as it was essential for him to achieve good daytime naps so he was not overtired at night. Oliver's most predictable daytime sleep was his morning nap around 10 a.m. We decided on a gradual retreat approach where Mum would settle him into his cot, sit on the floor at eye level (to encourage him to stay laying down rather than stand against the side of the cot) and to pat, soothe and make gentle shushing sounds. This obviously would involve crying as Oliver had never slept in a cot before so didn't know what was expected of him. I expected Oliver to resist sleeping, but reassured Mum that because she was staying with him at all times he would not feel abandoned as she was there to give him love and comfort, and she had a secure and strong attachment with him. For his health and well-being it was essential for him to learn the skill of self-settling in the safety of a cot. Mum was advised that she must see this process through until sleep was achieved and not give up otherwise she would be teaching him to cry for a fixed time. I advised that each time he fell asleep in this way, he would find it easier the next time. Every few days, Mum was to give less and less intervention with helping Oliver to sleep until she was eventually just sitting by his side and then she was to gradually move her chair away from the cot.

The next step was to reduce night-time feeds by cutting out feeds at particular times.

Outcome – Oliver responded very positively to not feeding to sleep as he still had Mum and/or Dad to lay down with him to begin with, so it was a very gradual withdrawal process. They slowly gave less and less intervention to help him get to sleep and this quickly resulted in him not waking during the early evening period when he was in his deep-sleep phase.

Helping him to sleep in a cot took a period of only 5 days. As expected, on day one, he stood up and cried a lot, but Mum stayed by his side and kept encouraging him to lay down and sleep, while soothing him. It took 1 hour of reassurance on the first day and then he slept soundly for 40 minutes. On day two, it took 35 minutes for him to get to sleep. On day three, his cries changed to protests and it took 55 minutes. Day 4, 30 minutes, again protesting, but not crying. On day five, it took only 5 minutes with no crying! Over time his naps became longer and he enjoyed going to sleep in his cot. Mum tended to stay with him until he went to sleep as this was her preference.

Oliver learnt very quickly to sleep in his cot and both his parents and I were very pleased with his response. I think this type of trust technique of staying with him suited the parenting style he was used to and he was also of an age where he understood what Mum was asking of him.

Interestingly, once he learnt to nap in his cot, when he was put in the parental bed in the evenings he pointed to his cot. His parents felt that this was his way of telling them he was ready for his own space, so he would start the evening in his cot and possibly end up in their bed if he fed in the night. This arrangement was an excellent compromise for all. He was sleeping well in the daytime and settling in his own cot in the evenings, so Mum and Dad could have an evening to themselves. He naturally started to wake less during the night for feeds as he was able to self-settle. It was a gradual gentle process that resulted in the whole family achieving better-quality sleep.

Mum's comments:
'Teaching Oliver to sleep in his cot has transformed our lives. My parents sometimes look after him when I am working and this now means he can have his daytime naps at their house. He has also happily slept in a travel cot while we were on holiday. In the early hours we still sometimes co-sleep too. Stephanie worked with us to provide a solution that suited us and our style of parenting and we are all now enjoying more sleep!'

Part Seven:
FURTHER RESOURCES AND INFORMATION

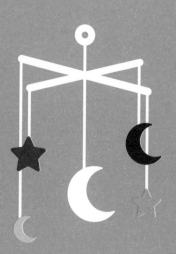

29. Sleep diary

Use your sleep diary to help you understand your baby's sleep patterns so you can determine how you need to regulate your daily feeding and napping routine.

	Time of last feed	Time started bath/ bed routine	Time baby went to bed	Time baby went to sleep
Monday				
Tuesday				
Wednesday				
Thursday				
Friday				
Saturday				
Sunday				

If your baby sleeps around the same time each day, they will find it easier to fall asleep. Try to avoid feeding just before a nap, as this will create a sleep association. The column below, for 'additional information', can include notes about outings, health, what worked well with regard to settling your baby, etc.

Time(s) baby woke in the night	What you did (i.e. fed, resettled with voice/touch)	Time woke in the morning	Additional Information/ nap times

30. Top sleep tips

When your baby is 3-6 months old, you can strongly influence when sleep occurs as babies respond well to routine and can differentiate between night and day. This is your window of opportunity to establish good sleep habits. Here are my top sleep tips. Keep them in a handy place, such as on the fridge door or at the front of your diary to refer to:

1. It's beneficial for babies over 3-4 months old to learn to fall asleep without any external props or associations. Props come in many forms and may include feeding to sleep by breast or bottle, rocking, cuddling, patting, music or a dummy. If your baby is reliant on one or more of these to fall asleep, they may need it each time they wake in between sleep cycles, which can be several times a night.

2. Encouraging your baby to learn to fall asleep independently is one of the most helpful things you can do to prevent or resolve settling and waking problems. Use a gradual retreat process if necessary.

3. At the start of the night, try to keep your baby awake while feeding and place them in their cot when they are drowsy but not asleep.

4. If your baby wakes during the night give them the opportunity to self-settle. Pause, listen and observe.

5. If you need to feed your baby during the night, have minimal interaction, only change their nappy if necessary and place them back in their cot straight after their feed, soothing as necessary.

6. Try to establish a positive sleep association – i.e. give your baby a safe, special soft toy or a soft cloth so this can become something they associate with sleep and that gives them comfort. Choose something that is safe and replaceable.

7. Establish a regular bedtime and morning wake-up time. This will regulate your baby's body clock and ensure healthy sleep/wake patterns. Aim for an early bedtime so your baby does not become overtired.

8. Create a predictable bedtime routine lasting no longer than 30–45 minutes. This might include quiet time, bath, pyjamas, feed, then maybe a short quiet story to make a break between feeding and sleeping to avoid creating an association. Alternatively, from around 4 months, consider giving the last feed before the bath.

9. Try to keep daytime naps and feeds regular and consistent. Again, do not feed to sleep. Try to time your feeds so that they are not just before a nap. Good daytime naps help good night-time sleeping, so don't be fooled into thinking that exhausting your baby and missing daytime naps will help them to sleep better at night. Just don't allow the last daytime nap to be too late and interfere with bedtime.

10. Let your baby have a voice! Don't try to immediately quell every cry. This is the only way for your baby to communicate with you, so in order for you to understand their needs, pause and listen, and try to learn to differentiate between their cries. Babies often grizzle themselves to sleep – this is normal.

11. If you are breastfeeding, try to avoid drinking caffeine, especially at the end of the day, and you may want to consider introducing an occasional bottle early enough to prevent later rejection. There are a number of breastfeeding-friendly bottles and teats available that emulate the breastfeeding process.

12. If your baby is still having regular night feeds at 6 months and is healthy and feeding well during the day, you can now begin to gradually wean them off these night feeds.

13. Be consistent! Whatever is happening at one sleep situation needs to be happening at all sleep situations to send a clear message about what is expected. This includes when your baby wakes during the night. If you occasionally take your baby into bed with you to sleep but expect them to sleep in their cot at other times they will become confused.

Remember, if you are making changes it takes **TIME**, **REPETITION** and **CONSISTENCY**.

14. Above all, enjoy your baby!

31. Useful organisations

The Lullaby Trust – www.lullabytrust.org.uk

NCT (National Childbirth Trust) – www.nct.org.uk

Baby Centre – www.babycentre.co.uk

Twins Trust – www.twinstrust.org

Basis (Baby Sleep Info Source) –
www.basisonline.org.uk

The Breastfeeding Network –
www.breastfeedingnetwork.org.uk

La Leche League (breastfeeding support) –
www.laleche.org.uk

Homestart – www.home-start.org.uk

Association for Post Natal Illness – www.apni.org

PaNDAS (PND Awareness and Support) –
www.pandasfoundation.org.uk

Cry-sis (support for parents with crying and sleepless
babies) – www.cry-sis.org.uk